The Natural Medicine Guide to

BIPOLAR
DISORDER

Stephanie Marohn

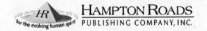 HAMPTON ROADS
PUBLISHING COMPANY, INC.

Cover design: Bookwrights Design
Cover art © 2002 Loyd Chapplow
Interior art by MediClip Images © 2003
Williams & Wilkins. All rights reserved.

Hampton Roads Publishing Company, Inc.
PO Box 8107
Charlottesville, VA 22906

434-296-2772
fax: 434-296-5096
e-mail: hrpc@hrpub.com
www.hrpub.com

If you are unable to order this book from your local
bookseller, you may order directly from the publisher.
Call 434-296-2772.

Library of Congress Cataloging-in-Publication Data

Marohn, Stephanie.
  The natural medicine guide to bipolar disorder /
Stephanie Marohn.
     p. ; cm. -- (The healthy mind guides)
Includes bibliographical references and index.
  ISBN 1-57174-291-3 (alk. paper)
  1. Manic-depressive illness--Alternative treatment.
  2. Naturopathy.
  [DNLM: 1. Bipolar Disorder--therapy--Popular Works.
  2. Homeopathy--Popular Works. 3. Naturopathy--Popular Works.
    WM 207 M354n
2003] I. Title. II. Series.
  RC516.M38 2003
  616.89'506--dc21

                                        2003001983

ISBN 978-1-57174-291-9
10 9 8 7
Printed on acid-free paper in Canada

THE HEALTHY MIND GUIDES

The Healthy Mind Guides are a series of books offering original research and treatment options for reversing or ameliorating several so-called mental disorders, written by noted health journalist and author Stephanie Marohn. The series' focus is the natural medicine approach, a refreshing and hopeful outlook based on treating individual needs rather than medical labels, and addressing the underlying imbalances—biological, psychological, emotional, and spiritual.

Each book in the series offers the very latest information about the possible causes of each disorder, and presents a wide range of effective, practical therapies drawn from extensive interviews with physicians and other practitioners who are innovators in their respective fields. Case studies throughout the books illustrate the applications of these therapies, and numerous resources are provided for readers who want to seek treatment.

♣

To Virginia Woolf

Contents

Acknowledgments

My deep gratitude to the doctors and other healing professionals who provided information on their work for the natural medicine treatment chapters in the book. I am very appreciative of all the time and energy you so generously gave. Specifically, my thanks to:

Lina Garcia, D.D.S., D.M.D.
Dietrich Klinghardt, M.D., Ph.D.
Devi S. Nambudripad, M.D., D.C., L.Ac., Ph.D.
Judyth Reichenberg-Ullman, N.D., L.C.S.W.
Julia Ross, M.A.
Malidoma Patrice Somé, Ph.D.
William J. Walsh, Ph.D.
Bradford S. Weeks, M.D.

Great thanks to my inspired physicians Dr. Ira Golchehreh and Dr. Thomas Rau for taking such good care of me.

Loving gratitude to my Gaia circle for being there through all the ups and downs of life.

Appreciation to Sue Trowbridge and Dorothy Anderson for all your hard work transcribing many interviews.

Continued and perpetual hosannas to my friend and editor Richard Leviton.

Thanks to all the staff at Hampton Roads.

Introduction

We in the United States and other countries in the developed world are in the midst of a mental health crisis. The psychiatric treatment methods we have been using are not working, as is clear from the dire statistics on mental illness. Here are just a few:

- Mental illness is the second leading cause of disability and premature mortality in the U.S. and other developed countries.[1]

- 4 of the 10 leading causes of disability in the U.S. and other developed countries are mental disorders—bipolar disorder, major depression, obsessive-compulsive disorder, or schizophrenia.[2]

- 5.4 percent of adults in the U.S. have a serious mental illness (defined as "substantial interference with one or more major life activities"; less severe mental illness is not included in this statistic).[3]

- 1 in 4 hospital admissions in the U.S. in 1998 were psychiatric admissions.[4]

- $148 billion = the total cost of mental illness in the U.S. in 1990 alone[5] ($69 billion in direct costs for mental health treatment and rehabilitation, and $79 billion in the indirect costs of lost productivity at work, school, or home due to disability or death).

A large reason why treatment of mental illness has a poor success record and is costing more all the time is that the overwhelming emphasis is placed on pharmaceutical drugs. Not everyone in the psychiatric field is happy with the ever-increasing governance of psychopharmacology (the science of drugs used to affect behavior and emotional states). Here is what one psychiatrist had to say about it. In December 1998, in a letter of resignation to the president of the American Psychiatric Association (APA), Loren R. Mosher, M.D., former official of the National Institute of Mental Health (NIMH), wrote:[6]

> "After nearly three decades as a member it is with a mixture of pleasure and disappointment that I submit this letter of resignation from the American Psychiatric Association. The major reason for this action is my belief that I am actually resigning from the American Psychopharmacological Association. . . .
>
> "At this point in history, in my view, psychiatry has been almost completely bought out by the drug companies. . . .
>
> "We condone and promote the widespread overuse and misuse of toxic chemicals that we know have serious long term effects . . . "

While psychiatric drugs (prescription drugs used for mental illnesses) may control certain disorders, and in some instances save lives, they do not cure the disorder, and they often compound the person's problems with disturbing side effects in the short term and the risk of permanent damage in the long term. If we are going to solve the current mental health crisis, we are going to have to turn to other approaches to treatment.

The state of affairs in psychiatric treatment is reflected in the focus of quite a few of the books on mental illness aimed at the general public. The help they offer involves information for the patient on coping with hospitalization; for family members on how to live with the illness in a loved one; and on how to work with side effects of psychopharmaceuticals (psychiatric drugs), that is, what other drugs you can take to reduce those effects.

The focus of *The Natural Medicine Guide to Bipolar Disorder* is healing from bipolar disorder (formerly known as manic-depression and characterized by often disabling mood swings), not learning how to endure it. The book explores the contributing factors and triggers and offers a range of treatment approaches to address them and truly restore health. Only by treating underlying imbalances, rather than suppressing the symptoms as most drugs do, can lasting recovery be achieved. And only by considering the well-being of the mind and spirit as well as the body can comprehensive healing take place.

The therapies covered in this book approach the treatment of bipolar disorder in this way. They all also share the characteristic of tailoring treatment to the individual, which is another essential element for a successful outcome. No two people, even with the same diagnosis, have exactly the same imbalances causing their problems.

With the increase in the number of people who are using natural therapies, the public has become more aware of this medical approach. When many people think of natural medicine, however, they think of supplements or herbal remedies available over the counter. While these products can be highly beneficial, natural medicine is far more than that.

Natural therapies are those that operate according to holistic principles, meaning treating the whole person rather than an isolated part or symptom and using natural treatments that "Do no harm" and support or restore the body's natural ability to heal itself. Natural medicine involves a way of looking at healing that is dramatically different from the conventional medical model. It does not mimic that model by merely substituting a nutritional supplement for a psychiatric drug. Instead, it is the comprehensive approach described above, which offers you the possibility of health.

Before I tell you a little about what's in the book, I have some comments about the terms "mental illness" and "mental disorders," or "brain disorders" as they are more currently labeled. All of these terms reflect the disconnection between body and mind—much less spirit—in conventional medical treatment. The newer term, brain disorders, reflects the biochemical model of causality that currently dominates the medical profession.

I use the terms "mental illness" and "mental disorders" in this book because there is no easy substitute that reflects the true body-mind-spirit nature of these conditions. While I may use these terms, I in no way mean to suggest that the causes of the disorders lie solely in the mind. The same is true for the title of the series of which this book is a part: The Healthy Mind Guides. The name serves to distinguish the subject area, but it is healthy mind, body, and spirit—wholeness—that is the focus of these books.

While I'm at it, I may as well dispense with one last linguistic issue. As natural medicine effects profound healing, rather than simply controlling symptoms, I prefer the term "natural medicine" over "alternative medicine." This medical model is not "other"—it is a primary form of medicine. The term "holistic medicine" reflects this as well, in that it signals the natural medicine approach of treating the whole person, rather than the parts.

As I said, the focus of this book is on comprehensive treatments. While there are a number of natural self-help medicines that can be useful in alleviating mild or moderate depression or anxiety associated with bipolar disorder, they do not address the underlying causes and, for that reason, I don't cover them in this book, which is dedicated to the deeper treatments. In addition, bipolar states are often on the severe end of the mood spectrum and require care beyond self-help. (For self-help treatments for depression and anxiety, see my book *Natural Medicine First Aid Remedies,* Hampton Roads, 2001.)

Part I of *The Natural Medicine Guide to Bipolar Disorder* covers the basics of bipolar disorder: what it is, who gets it, and what causes it. The natural medicine view is that it is a multicausal disorder, with a variety of contributing factors.

Part II of the book covers a range of natural medicine treatments for bipolar disorder. The material presented here is based on research and interviews with physicians and other healing professionals who are leaders and pioneers in their respective fields.

This is original information, not derivative material gleaned from secondary sources. The therapeutic techniques of these highly skilled and experienced healers are explained in detail and illustrated with case studies (the names of patients throughout the book have been changed). Contact information for the practitioners whose work is presented appears in appendix B: Resources.

May the information in this book help you recover from bipolar disorder and find your way to greater mood stability.

Natural Medicine Therapies
Covered in Part II

Chapter	Health Practitioner	Therapies/Testing
3	Dietrich Klinghardt, M.D., Ph.D.	APN (applied psychoneurobiology) Chelation/heavy metal detoxification Family Systems Therapy Neural therapy
4	Bradford S. Weeks, M.D.	Biological medicine Anthroposophic medicine
5	William J. Walsh, Ph.D.	Biochemical therapy Urine and blood testing Metallothionein dysfunction therapy
6	Julia Ross, M.A.	Amino acid/nutritional therapy
7	Lina Garcia, D.D.S., D.M.D.	Cranial osteopathy Family Systems Therapy
8	Devi S. Nambudripad, M.D., D.C., L.Ac., Ph.D.	NAET (allergy testing and elimination; includes MRT, muscle response testing)
9	Judyth Reichenberg-Ullman, N.D., L.C.S.W.	Constitutional homeopathy
10	Malidoma Patrice Somé, Ph.D.	Shamanic healing

PART I

The Basics of Bipolar Disorder

1 What Is Bipolar Disorder and Who Suffers from It?

The often outrageous, flamboyant behavior associated with the manic pole of bipolar disorder has garnered both media attention and public fascination, but many people remain unaware of the painful, debilitating, and devastating aspects of the illness—on both ends of the mood spectrum.

While a stressful event may trigger an episode, often the mood swings of bipolar disorder are inexplicable, bearing no apparent relation to what is happening in a person's life. Far beyond happy or sad moods, the condition is often agonizing and even life threatening. It wreaks havoc in careers, relationships, lives.

The medical and psychiatric professions classify bipolar disorder as a mental illness, and more specifically, as a mood disorder, or affective disorder. The psychiatric and medical professions regard bipolar disorder as a biological brain condition, which has a genetic basis and involves disturbed brain chemistry. Formerly known as manic-depression, it is characterized by periods of depression and mania, with wide variation in the length, frequency, severity, and fluctuation of these periods. Each episode can last days or months and there may or may not be intervals of normal mood states between episodes. When there are such intervals, they can extend to days, months, or even many years.

Mania is characterized by an elevated, expansive, or irritable and angry mood with increased activity and energy, thought, and

3

speech that is more rapid than usual, reduced need for sleep, grandiosity, distractibility, impulsiveness, inflated self-esteem, poor judgment, and/or recklessness, as in questionable sexual behavior and lavish spending sprees. In extreme episodes, delusions or hallucinations can occur.

Episodes of depression are characterized by persistent sadness or a feeling of flatness, pessimism, hopelessness, significantly reduced interest or pleasure, significant change in weight or appetite, insomnia or oversleeping, feelings of worthlessness or excessive or inappropriate guilt, problems thinking, concentrating, or making decisions, lethargy or restlessness and agitation, lack of energy, and/or recurrent thoughts of death or suicide. Delusions, and less often, hallucinations, can occur in depressive episodes as well as in manic.

While the name bipolar disorder reflects two distinct mood poles, the separation of mania and depression in this way is misleading in regard to what many people who suffer from the disorder actually experience, which is often an overlapping, mixed mood state. For this reason, Kay Redfield Jamison, Ph.D., an authority on the disorder and a person who suffered from it from the age of 17, prefers the former name, manic-depression, as more accurately descriptive. "This polarization of two clinical states flies in the face of everything that we know about the cauldronous, fluctuating nature of manic-depressive illness; it ignores the question of whether mania is, ultimately, simply an extreme form of depression; and it minimizes the importance of mixed manic-and-depressive states, conditions that are common . . ."[7]

Bipolar disorder tends to run in families and usually manifests in late adolescence or early adulthood, but onset can also occur during preteen and later adult years. The peak age of onset is the mid-twenties,[8] although that average may be dropping as more young children are developing the disorder (see "Children and Bipolar Disorder," which follows). While there is no one pattern of progression in bipolar disorder, when untreated, it tends over time to escalate both in frequency and severity of episodes.

Unfortunately, only one in three people with a major mood disorder seek help.[9] Many people are not aware that they are suffer-

Facts about Bipolar Disorder

- 2.3 million adults in the United States have bipolar disorder.

- An estimated 1 million children under the age of 18 in the United States have bipolar disorder.

- The onset of bipolar disorder in nearly half of those who suffer from it occurred before they were 21; for 1 in 5 the onset occurred in childhood.

- While depression affects twice as many women as men, bipolar disorder affects men and women equally.

- While rates of depression vary greatly from country to country, rates of bipolar disorder are relatively consistent across countries.

- 90 percent of people with bipolar disorder have a close relative who suffers from a mood disorder.

- Having one bipolar parent gives a child a 10 percent to 30 percent chance of becoming bipolar; with two bipolar parents, the risk can be as high as 75 percent.

- Among people with bipolar disorder, the rate of alcoholism and drug abuse is three times that of the general population.

- As many as 1 in 5 people with bipolar disorder will commit suicide.[10]

ing from bipolar disorder and so do not seek treatment. Even if they do, they may not get a proper diagnosis. There is no test for bipolar disorder and diagnosis is based largely on family history and the patient's pattern of mood swings. It is not unusual for people to endure the emotional roller coaster of bipolar disorder for a decade or more (the average is eight years between onset and diagnosis[11]) before a particularly bad episode finally results in a

Children and Bipolar Disorder

More children are now being diagnosed with bipolar disorder. An estimated one million children under the age of 18 now suffer from the condition. Among the reasons cited for the rise of the disorder among youth is an increase in childhood triggers, notably earlier drug use (particularly cocaine, amphetamines, and other stimulants) and higher stress levels at home and school. Some researchers postulate that "something in the environment" may be providing the trigger (see chapter 2 for a discussion of toxins). Improved diagnostic practices may also be a factor in reports of rising incidence among children.

With misdiagnosis a large problem, however, the number of children who are bipolar is likely even higher than the estimated one million. As many as 15 percent of children diagnosed with ADHD and almost 50 percent of those diagnosed with depression may actually be bipolar. Unfortunately, Ritalin and antidepressants, the drugs used to treat those conditions, can trigger or deepen a bipolar episode.[12]

diagnosis and subsequent treatment. Sadly, suicide claims many people before they get the help they need.

Bipolar disorder can be a corollary of other medical conditions such as an underactive thyroid (see chapter 2), and there is a comorbidity factor with substance abuse, obsessive-compulsive disorder, and panic disorder.[13] *Comorbidity* means that two disorders exist together. In the case of substance abuse, more than 60 percent of people with bipolar disorder abuse drugs or alcohol.[14] While the motivation may be self-medication to numb the pain of depression or calm the agitation of mania, in the case of alcohol, and to increase or induce the high of mania or attempt to lift depression, in the case of stimulants such as cocaine and amphetamines, the combination of bipolar disorder and substance abuse worsens the outcome of the illness. Those who abuse substances tend to have the irritable and paranoid, rather than the elated, type of mania, are more at risk for relapse, are more at risk for lithium not working for them, and experience 50 percent more hospitalizations.[15] Alcohol abuse also increases the likelihood of suicide, as alcohol features in 30 percent of all suicides.[16]

Nearly one in five people with bipolar disorder commit suicide.[17] The growing number of children with bipolar disorder may be a factor in the rising suicide rate among America's young. Suicide among the teen population has increased 300 percent in the past 30 years.[18] Among children between the ages of 10 and 14, the rate of suicide has more than doubled in the last ten years. For youth between the ages of 15 and 24, suicide is now the third leading cause of death. For college students, it is the second leading cause.[19] Note that in almost half of those with bipolar disorder, onset came before they were 21 years old. As the cycling of moods in bipolar children tends to be "ultra-rapid," with several mood changes in the space of a day,[20] you can imagine how difficult that makes life for these children.

The high incidence of suicide among people with bipolar disorder makes it important for both those with the condition as well as their family and friends to be aware of the warning signs of suicide. Being forewarned may enable you to prevent this tragedy from happening if the signs begin to manifest. A family history of suicide or a previous suicide attempt places one at increased risk of suicide. In addition, the warning signs of suicide are:[21]

- feelings of hopelessness, worthlessness, anguish, or desperation
- withdrawal from people and activities
- preoccupation with death or morbid subjects
- sudden mood improvement or increased activity after a period of depression
- increase in risk-taking behaviors
- buying a gun
- putting affairs in order
- thinking, talking, or writing about a plan for committing suicide.

If you think that you or someone you know is in danger of attempting suicide, call your doctor or a suicide hotline or get help from another qualified source. Know that there is help and, though it may be difficult to ask for it, a life may depend upon it.

Types of Bipolar Disorder

The numerous variations in the manifestation of bipolar disorder are reflected in the complicated array of psychiatric labels that fall under the heading of bipolar disorder. Further, the clinical status of a given episode can be specified as mild, moderate, or severe, with or without psychotic features, chronic, with rapid cycling, with catatonic features, or with melancholic features, among others.[22]

The following are subcategories of the bipolar psychiatric label, according to the diagnostic bible of the psychiatric profession, the *DSM-IV-TR (Diagnostic and Statistical Manual of Mental Disorders, Fourth Edition, Text Revision)*.[23] A holistic medical approach does not use such diagnoses to determine the appropriate treatment course, focusing instead on the particular manifestations and underlying imbalances in the individual patient. Many people receive these labels, however, so it's helpful to know to what they refer.

Bipolar Disorder I

In simple terms, Bipolar Disorder I ranges the whole spectrum from severe depression to mania or mixed mania, with an emphasis on the manic end. In *DSM-IV* terms, diagnosis requires that the person has had one or more manic episodes or mixed episodes (see list), and often has had one or more major depressive episodes in addition. The average age of onset in men and women alike is 20 years old for this form of bipolar disorder.[24]

A manic episode is defined as an abnormally elevated, expansive, or irritable mood persisting for at least one week (less if hospitalization ensues) and accompanied by at least three (four in the case of irritability only) of the following symptoms:[25]

- inflated self-esteem or grandiosity
- reduced need for sleep
- increased or more continual talking than usual
- flight of ideas, racing thoughts
- distractibility
- increased activity and energy or agitation
- excessive engagement in high-consequence activities such as unrestrained shopping, foolish business investments, and questionable sexual liaisons.

The mood alteration must also be severe enough to impair the person's functioning professionally, socially, or in relationships with others. The mania may also have psychotic features and/or require hospitalization. Paranoia may be part of the symptom picture.

A major depressive episode is defined as depressed mood or loss of interest lasting at least two weeks and accompanied by at least four of the following symptoms:[26]

- persistent sadness
- significantly reduced interest or pleasure
- significant change in weight or appetite
- insomnia or oversleeping
- restlessness, agitation, or lethargy
- fatigue or lack of energy
- feelings of worthlessness or excessive or inappropriate guilt
- problems thinking, concentrating, or making decisions
- recurrent thoughts of death or suicide.

When only major depressive episodes occur, without episodes of mania, the person is said to suffer from unipolar depression, also known as clinical depression.

For information about unipolar depression, see the author's *The Natural Medicine Guide to Depression* (Hampton Roads, 2003).

Bipolar Disorder II

Research suggests that this form of bipolar is more common than Bipolar Disorder I in general, and it appears to be more common among women. Bipolar Disorder II favors the depressive end of the mood spectrum, ranging from severe depression to hypomania (mild mania). Interestingly, men tend to experience as many or more hypomanic episodes as major depressive episodes, while for women the latter are more prevalent.[27] For a diagnosis of Bipolar Disorder II, according to the *DSM-IV,* the person must have had one or more major depressive episodes and one or more hypomanic episodes, never had a manic episode or a mixed episode, and had the disturbance impair, or produce distress in, the person's professional, social, or other important functioning.[28]

Hypomania is the same as mania, except the altered mood must last at least four days (rather than a week) and does not impair professional or social functioning, require hospitalization, or have psychotic features.

Cyclothymic Disorder

Cyclothymia ranges from mild or moderate depression (dysthymia) to hypomania. According to *DSM-IV* criteria for the diagnosis of cyclothymic disorder, the person must have had numerous periods of both hypomanic and depressive symptoms over at least two years, with no more than two months at a time free of symptoms, and with no major depressive episode, manic episode, or mixed episode during the first two years.

Mixed Episode

A mixed episode, also called a mixed state, mixed affective state, mixed mania, or dysphoric mania, is a manifestation of bipolar disorder in which depression and mania exist together in one episode. The *DSM-IV* defines it as a period of at least a week during which the person fits the picture for both a manic episode and a major depressive episode, with agitation, insomnia, psychotic features, and suicidal ideation often present.[29]

Rapid Cycling, Ultra-Rapid Cycling

This refers to a pattern that can occur in Bipolar I and Bipolar II. In rapid cycling, the moods are the same as defined, but they change more frequently, with four or more episodes in the space of a year, marked by a switch to the other pole or a period of nonepisodic mood (neither mania nor depression). Ultra-rapid cycling, a relatively new term, refers to switching that happens in the space of a day or even from moment to moment.

> ## In Their Own Words
>
> *"On occasion, these periods of total despair would be made even worse by terrible agitation. My mind would race from subject to subject, but instead of being filled with the exuberant and cosmic thoughts that had been associated with earlier periods of rapid thinking, it would be drenched in awful sounds and images of decay and dying."[30]*
> —Kay Redfield Jamison, Ph.D., on mixed episodes

Schizoaffective Disorder

While this disorder is listed under schizophrenia in the *DSM-IV*, it is defined as involving a major depressive, manic, or mixed episode in combination with two or more of the characteristic symptoms of schizophrenia: delusions, hallucinations, disorganized speech, catatonic or grossly disorganized behavior, or negative symptoms such as flat affect, lack of speech, or lack of volition. Schizoaffective disorder presents very much like bipolar disorder with psychotic features, the difference being that delusions and hallucinations in the latter case are part of the abnormal mood, while no such relationship exists in schizoaffective disorder.[31]

People with bipolar disorder are frequently diagnosed with schizophrenia and vice versa. Others receive a dual diagnosis of schizophrenia and bipolar disorder, as was true with several of the people featured in cases in this book. The schizoaffective category

In Their Own Words

"As with many people, the overt symptoms of my manic-depressive illness didn't show themselves until my late teens. . . . From that time on, until I was diagnosed at the age of 35, I rode a wild roller coaster, from agitated, out-of-control highs to disabling, often suicidal lows."[32]

—Patty Duke, actor and author of several books on manic-depression

highlights the confusion in attempting to distinguish between the disorders.

Bipolar Disorder and Creativity

There is another side to bipolar disorder, and that is its link to creativity. Madness in general has long been paired with genius in the arts. Investigation reveals that there is some substance behind what some dismiss as a romantic notion. Many people with bipolar disorder report that their creative output increases significantly when they are hypomanic. Researchers have cited "sharpened and unusually creative thinking" and "increased productivity" as two of the criteria in the diagnosis of hypomania.[33]

As part of her investigation into the relationship between creativity and mood disorders, Dr. Jamison charted the works of composer Robert Schumann in relation to his bipolar episodes, and the results are significant. During the years in which he was severely depressed or attempted suicide, he produced no, or one to two, opuses. In 1840 and 1849, when he was hypomanic for the whole year, he composed 24 and 27 opuses, respectively.[34]

There seems to be a preponderance of the affliction in artists and writers throughout history who were known to have mood disorders of some kind. This perception is borne out by a review of studies investigating the actual percentages in comparison with the population at large. An analysis of seven studies found that the rate of manic-depression and cyclothymia among artists and writers is 10 to 20 times higher than the rate in the general population; the rate of depression is 8 to 10 times higher; and the suicide rate is as much as 18 times higher.[35]

It is not known why this is so. Does the artistic process promote madness, or are people suffering from mental illness temperamentally drawn to the arts? Whatever the reason for the greater incidence among the creative, it is important not to lose sight of the tragic aspect of the madness-genius equation, which can get lost in the romanticization of the artistic life. As Dr. Jamison observes, "No one is creative when paralytically depressed, psychotic, institutionalized, in restraints, or dead because of suicide."[36]

The relationship between creativity and at least the milder form of mania makes treatment problematic for some people. The most common side effects that people on lithium report are "mental slowing" and "impaired concentration."[37] This is enough for some people to stop taking lithium. While avoiding the more debilitating form of mania may be an incentive for treatment compliance, hypomania may be a compelling state. As Dr. Jamison poses it, "Who would *not* want an illness that has among its symptoms elevated and expansive mood, inflated self-esteem, abundance of energy, less need for sleep, intensified sexuality, . . . sharpened and unusually creative thinking and increased productivity?"[38]

The relationship between creativity and at least the milder form of mania makes treatment problematic for some people. The most common side effects that people on lithium report are "mental slowing" and "impaired concentration." This is enough for some people to stop taking lithium.

It may not be only the hypomanic aspect of bipolar disorder that has an effect on creativity, "but rather the flux and tensions between the different mood states," explains psychiatrist and author Francis Mark Mondimore, M.D. "Perhaps bipolar disorder stimulates creativity in part because its sufferers experience the world through the emotional prisms of its many and shifting moods . . ."[39]

Famous People with Bipolar Disorder

The following are among the well-known people with bipolar disorder:[40]

Hector Berlioz	Margot Kidder
John Berryman	Henry James
William Blake	Charles Lamb
Napolean Bonaparte	Robert Lowell
Lord Byron	Gustav Mahler
Winston Churchill	Herman Melville
Kurt Cobain	Edgar Allan Poe
Samuel Taylor Coleridge	Theodore Roethke
William Cowper	Robert Schumann
Patty Duke	Anne Sexton
F. Scott Fitzgerald	Percy Bysshe Shelley
Graham Greene	Vincent van Gogh
George Frideric Handel	Tennessee Williams
Ernest Hemingway	Virginia Woolf

The Medical History of Bipolar Disorder

Mood disorders have plagued humankind for at least as long as recorded history, and likely from the beginning of human existence. Written accounts of mood disorders come to us from Egypt in the time of the pharaohs, 4,000 years ago.[41] Writings by physicians in ancient Greece describe both melancholia (a term for depression) and mania. One in particular, Aretaeus of Cappadocia, writing in around 150 A.D., expressed an understanding of the interrelationship of the two, as in bipolar disorder: "In my opinion, melancholia is without any doubt the beginning and even part of the disorder called mania."[42]

One way of explaining the presence of mood in the human spirit is to regard it as an evolutionary adaptation.[43] A depression in mood, for example, pulls us back from engagement with life, which we may need at that moment to keep us safe or to give us time to gain a perspective, while mania gives us the wherewithal to act quickly. Psychiatrist and author Peter C. Whybrow, M.D., suggests, "Perhaps mania and melancholia endure because they coexist with behaviors that serve a greater human purpose, attributes that have had survival value for the individual and thus, indirectly, are useful to society."[44]

In ancient Greece, melancholy came to be considered an excess of black bile, one of the four "humors" of the body (blood, black bile, yellow bile, and phlegm) believed to regulate health. According to humoral theory, as suggested by one physician, mania was the result of too much yellow bile that had turned into black bile as a consequence of too much heat.[45] Black bile was considered the driving force in creativity, so melancholy gained a positive association with the creative temperament. By pointing out the many poets, artists, politicians, Greek heroes, and philosophers, including Plato and Socrates, who were of a melancholic nature, Aristotle perpetuated a positive view of the condition that continued for centuries.[46]

In the Middle Ages, mental illnesses came to be viewed as conditions to cure, with demonic possession or witchcraft their cause. During this period, priests delivered the exorcistic ministrations that were considered treatment.

Although the mania and depression of bipolar disorder was first described as one mental illness in 1854, by two French physicians, a full description did not appear until 1899 in a textbook by German physician Emil Kraepelin.[47] He studied and documented bipolar disorder and other mental illnesses, providing the foundation for modern psychiatry, whose focus on diagnosis and classification comes from Dr. Kraepelin.[48]

The belief that psychological factors were the cause of mental illnesses arose from the work of Sigmund Freud and began to gain cachet in the American medical establishment in the 1920s.[49] With the source of such illness firmly placed in the mind, parents (mostly mothers), early trauma, and psychological conflicts became the culprits behind manic-depression and schizophrenia. This orientation is largely responsible for the stigma that came to be attached to mental illness—that is, manic-depression is not a disease like any other, but a failing on the part of the individual or the individual's mother.

The advent of psychiatric drugs in the 1950s transformed the psychiatric field, shifting the focus of the causality of mental illness from psychological to biochemical, and turning the profession into a pharmaceutical industry. Gradually, the medical redefinition with its focus on biology permeated public consciousness, but the stigma attached to mental illness persists to a certain degree, although open discussion by celebrities suffering from the disorder has helped dispel some of the earlier judgments and misconceptions. Medically, the role of psychological factors in bipolar disorder is not entirely discounted, but the overwhelming emphasis in treatment is on drugs.

The Pharmacological Age

The current conventional medical view is that bipolar disorder is a brain disorder involving some kind of neurotransmitter malfunction. Neurotransmitters are the brain's chemical messengers that enable communication between cells. While there are many different kinds of neurotransmitters, the primary ones involved in the regulation of mood are serotonin, dopamine, epinephrine/norepinephrine, GABA (gamma-aminobutyric acid), and L-glutamate.

Contrary to popular belief, serotonin is not found only in the brain. In fact, only 5 percent of the body's supply is in the brain, with 95 percent distributed throughout the body and involved in many functions.[50]

Serotonin is distributed throughout the brain, where it is "the single largest brain system known."[51]

In addition to influencing mood, serotonin is involved in the regulation of sleep and pain, to name but a few of its numerous activities.

Dopamine has a role in controlling sex drive, memory retrieval, and muscles, as well as mood. One theory holds that dopamine may be operating to excess in severe mania and acute schizophrenia.[53]

GABA operates to stop excess nerve stimulation, thereby exerting a calming effect on the brain. Two important functions of L-glutamate involve memory and the curbing of chronic stress response and excess secretion of the adrenal "stress" hormone cortisol.

Epinephrine (also known as adrenaline) and norepinephrine are hormones produced by the adrenal gland. Epinephrine is involved in the stress response and the physiology of fear and anxiety; an excess has been implicated in some anxiety disorders. Norepinephrine is similar to epinephrine and is the form of adrenaline found in the brain;[54] interference with norepinephrine metabolism at certain brain sites has been linked to affective disorders.[55]

> **In Their Own Words**
>
> *"You move seamlessly through something wonderful to the plausible, although far-fetched, to ideas and thoughts that are completely implausible, before sliding into a self-deluded confusion."*[52]
>
> —Stephan Szabo, on his experience of mania

Neurotransmitters are the targets of psychiatric drugs used in the treatment of mental illness. In the case of bipolar disorder, these drugs fall into the categories of mood stabilizers (lithium and anti-convulsant drugs), antipsychotics, antidepressants, and tranquilizers. While the effects and side effects of all could be enumerated at length, the following brief discussion focuses on a few of the drugs in the first three categories typically used in bipolar disorder.

Although the application of the chemical lithium (with the addition of the compound carbonate it becomes lithium salts) in bipolar disorder was discovered in the late 1940s, the U.S. Food and Drug Administration (FDA) did not approve it for preventive use in bipolar disorder until 1974. After that, it became standard drug treatment. Lithium works by affecting neurotransmitters in some way to slow the electrical transmission of brain cells, which impedes the person's ability to feel or react.

"Lithium flattens emotions by blunting or constricting the range of feeling, resulting in varying degrees of apathy and indifference," state Peter R. Breggin, M.D., and David Cohen, Ph.D., authors of *Your Drug May Be Your Problem*. "It also slows down the thinking processes. This drug-induced mental and emotional sluggishness should be considered lithium's primary 'therapeutic' effect."[56]

There is no doubt that the advent of lithium saved, and continues to save, many lives. At the same time, there are a number of reasons to consider alternatives. Lithium produces no effect in 30 percent of people with bipolar disorder and others cannot tolerate the side effects.[57] A summary of data on adverse drug effects found that 32.5 percent of patients on lithium experienced memory impairment, and 22.8 percent (in some studies the rate was almost 40 percent) experienced confusion and disorientation.[58] For some patients, discontinuing lithium treatment does not lead to a restoration of full mental function; in other words, effects can be permanent. In addition, lithium can cause hypothyroidism, among other conditions. Withdrawal from the drug can trigger a manic episode.

"Lithium flattens emotions by blunting or constricting the range of feeling, resulting in varying degrees of apathy and indifference," state Peter R. Breggin, M.D., and David Cohen, Ph.D., authors of Your Drug May Be Your Problem. "It also slows down the thinking processes. This drug-induced mental and emotional sluggishness should be considered lithium's primary 'therapeutic' effect."

Even a recent article in the *Journal of Clinical Psychiatry* on the use of lithium for bipolar disorder concluded: "Lithium is the only agent currently approved for the treatment of both acute episodes of mania and maintenance therapy; however, it is associated with a relatively poor response rate, high relapse rate, and less-than-optimal side effect profile."[59]

Like lithium, anticonvulsants are used as mood stabilizers. Perhaps the most well known in the treatment of bipolar disorder is Depakote, which was originally used for epilepsy. It is not known how these drugs work to control mania or reduce mood swings. Known side effects of Depakote are sedation, confusion, impairment of mental function, tremors, walking problems, and even delirium.[60]

Antipsychotics such as Thorazine have a history of use in mental illness, including bipolar disorder. Also known as neuroleptics (the literal translation is "taking hold of the nerves"), and formerly referred to as major tranquilizers, these drugs blunt a range of brain activities and produce "apathy, indifference, emotional blandness, conformity, and submissiveness, as well as a reduction in all verbalizations, including complaints or protests," according to Drs. Breggin and Cohen. "It is no exaggeration to call this effect a chemical lobotomy," they state.[61]

The phrase "the Thorazine shuffle" came into usage in mental hospitals in the early days of Thorazine prescription, referring to the characteristic way of moving as a result of the numbing physical, mental, and emotional effects of this drug.

Although antipsychotics are ostensibly given to control delusions and hallucinations, they actually have no specific effects on either, say Drs. Breggin and Cohen, and their side effects are daunting. While so-called atypical antipsychotics, such as Zyprexa, are enjoying cachet now over Thorazine and other typical antipsychotics because their side effects are regarded as less onerous, Drs. Breggin and Cohen strongly state: "All neuroleptics produce an enormous variety of

Prescription Drugs Commonly Used to Control Bipolar Disorder
Antidepressants
Celexa (citalopram)
Desyrel (trazodone)
Paxil (paroxetine)
Prozac (fluoxetine)
Wellbutrin (bupropion)
Zoloft (sertraline)
Antipsychotics (typical)
Haldol (haloperidol)
Thorazine (chlorpromazine)
Antipsychotics (atypical)
Clozaril (clozapine)
Risperdal (risperidone)
Zyprexa (olanzapine)
Mood stabilizers
Depakote (divalproex sodium)
Lamictal (lamotrigine)
lithium carbonate
Tegretol (carbamazepine)
Topamax (topiramate)
Tranquilizers
Ativan (lorazepam)
Klonopin (clonazepam)
Valium (diazepam)

potentially severe and disabling neurological impairments at extraordinarily high rates of occurrence; they are among the most toxic agents ever administered to people."[62]

Meanwhile, more and more children are being diagnosed with bipolar disorder and put on antipsychotics.

Antidepressants target serotonin, dopamine, and norepinephrine, which are monoamines (they are derived from amino acids) colloquially known as the "feel good" neurotransmitters.[63] The antidepressant drugs Prozac, Paxil, Zoloft, Luvox, and Effexor are what is known as SSRIs, selective serotonin re-uptake inhibitors. They block the natural reabsorption of serotonin by brain cells, which boosts the level of available serotonin. SSRIs are relatively new arrivals on the antidepressant scene; Prozac was introduced on the market in 1987.

Earlier categories of antidepressant drugs are tricyclics and monoamine oxidase inhibitors (MAOIs). Tricyclics such as Elavil, Adapin, and Endep inhibit serotonin re-uptake, but block norepinephrine re-uptake as well; thus, they are less selective than SSRIs. MAOIs such as Nardil and Parnate act by inhibiting a certain MAO enzyme that breaks down monoamines; the outcome is more available neurotransmitters.[64]

The theory that neurotransmitter deficiency causes depression is known as the "biogenic amine" hypothesis. While the model recognizes that imbalances in amino acids (neurotransmitter precursors) produce the deficiency, amino acid supplementation is not the conventional medical solution. "These amino acids have proven to be effective natural antidepressants," states Michael T. Murray, N.D., author of *Natural Alternatives to Prozac.*[65] Despite this, the focus of conventional treatment is expensive pharmaceuticals. "Perhaps the main reason [the biogenic amine] model is so popular is that it is a better fit for drug therapy," notes Dr. Murray.[66]

 For more about amino acids, see chapters 5 and 6.

Contrary to popular belief, the newer, more expensive antidepressants—Prozac, Zoloft, and Paxil—are no more effective than the older antidepressant drugs, according to a report issued by researchers for the U.S. Agency for Health Care Policy and Research and the U.S. Department of Health and Human Services.[67]

In disregard of disturbing side effects and of research showing that they do not work for a third of the people who take them, and do no better than placebos for another third,[68] these drugs continue to be dispensed widely and to be regarded as the panacea for depression. This prescription flurry is extending to children now as well. With the growing number of children being diagnosed with bipolar disorder, more children are being put on antidepressants, despite the fact that Prozac and similar antidepressants are approved by the FDA only for use in patients over the age of 18.[69]

The adverse effects (euphemistically known as side effects) of antidepressants can range from uncomfortable to untenable, although some people who take the drugs experience no side effects. With Prozac, for example, adverse effects include nausea, headaches, anxiety and nervousness, insomnia, drowsiness, diarrhea, dry mouth, loss of appetite, sweating and tremor, and rash.[70]

Flattened or dulled feelings and sexual dysfunction are common effects of taking SSRIs. In addition, the anxiety and agitation induced by SSRIs can result in patients increasing their use of alcohol and other substances for calming purposes.[71]

More serious, there has been very little research on the long-term effects of taking SSRIs. It is known, however, that they can produce neurological disorders, and permanent brain damage is a danger.[72]

Of particular importance to people with bipolar disorder is the fact that antidepressants can not only trigger a manic episode, but can also accelerate the illness, plunging the person into more frequent mood changes and even rapid cycling,[73]

This is something that the psychiatric profession has known about since the 1950s. Both the older antidepressants and their newer relatives, the SSRIs, are linked to this phenomenon. Since more people are now taking antidepressants than ever before, this puts more people at risk. One study found that the mania or psychosis of 43 out of 533 patients admitted to a psychiatric hospital was connected to antidepressant use, and 70 percent of those patients were on Prozac, Zoloft, Paxil, or another SSRI.[74]

While this drug reaction does not occur in everyone with bipolar disorder, it is unknown who is at risk. Those who are aware that they have bipolar disorder can at least be forewarned that this is a possibility, but people who do not know that they have the condition and seek treatment for depression can suffer serious consequences. This is why it is so important for physicians, before prescribing antidepressants, to take full medical histories, including inquiring into a patient's past mood patterns and whether there is a history of mood disorders in the family.

In addition to the range of drugs cited, more drugs are often prescribed to counteract the side effects of the others. The result is that many people with bipolar disorder are on a kind of drug "cocktail," a mixture of quite a few medications. Most face a lifetime of this because these drugs are not a cure, but only a means of controlling the symptoms, and often not well at that. There is no doubt that lithium and antidepressants save lives, but they do not address the underlying factors that cause or contribute to the condition, even the most fundamental factor of nutritional deficiencies that lead to an imbalance in amino acids and neurotransmitters. Investigation into these factors is rarely a feature in drug-based treatment.

Natural medicine is based on the knowledge that in order for comprehensive healing to occur, the factors causing or contributing to a disorder must be identified and addressed in each person. With this approach, it is possible for people to get off their drugs or reduce their dosages, and in so doing improve their present and future health. The next chapter explores the underlying factors that can play a role in bipolar disorder.

2 Causes, Triggers, and Contributors

The cause of bipolar disorder is unknown, beyond a general belief that there is an as yet unidentified genetic component. As with other "mental" illnesses, it appears that environmental factors combine with genetic vulnerability to trigger the disorder. Science does not know what impels the episodic shifts once bipolar disorder has developed, as they often occur independent of obvious influences.

The reality is that, in spite of their widespread acceptance in the medical community, the disease model that resulted in the classification of bipolar disorder and schizophrenia as mental illnesses, the genetic component, and the focus on neurotransmitter dysfunction as the source of the problem are all suspect.

Here is what some eminent psychiatrists and researchers had to say on the subject:

> "[T]here is no proven physical cause for any psychiatric disorder . . . [W]hy are so many . . . convinced that the origins of mental illnesses are to be found in biology, when, despite more than three decades of research, there is still no proof? . . . The absence of any well-defined physical causation is reflected in the absence of any laboratory tests for psychiatric diagnoses—much in contrast to diabetes and many other physical disorders."
> —Charles E. Dean, M.D., director of psychiatric residency at the Minneapolis Veterans Medical Center, quoted in the *Minnesota Star Tribune* (November 22, 1997).[75]

"Contrary to what is often claimed, no biochemical, anatomical or functional signs have been found that reliably distinguish the brains of mental patients."

—Dr. Elliot Valenstein, Ph.D., University of
Michigan neuroscientist and professor emeritus
of psychology, author of *Blaming the Brain:
The Truth About Drugs and Mental Health*.[76]

"[W]e have no identified etiological agents for psychiatric disorders."

—Gary J. Tucker, M.D., professor and chairman
of psychiatry and behavioral sciences at the University
of Washington School of Medicine, quoted in the
American Journal of Psychiatry (February 1998).[77]

"Through the 1970s and 1980s, a curious circularity invaded psychiatry, as 'diseases' began to be 'modeled' on the medications that 'treat' them. If a drug elevated serotonin in test tubes, then it was presumptuously argued that patients helped by the medication must have serotonin deficiencies even though we lack scientific proof for the idea."

—Joseph Glenmullen, M.D., clinical instructor
in psychiatry at Harvard Medical School
and author of *Prozac Backlash*.[78]

From a holistic viewpoint, a single physiological cause or even one such cause in combination with a genetic abnormality is not the sum total of a condition such as bipolar disorder. Perhaps research has been unable to identify an "etiological agent" because "mental illness" is the outcome of body-mind-spirit disturbance caused by physical, psychological, emotional, spiritual, and energetic influences, each of which affects all of the other areas so no influence can be considered in isolation.

If we acknowledge that body, mind, and spirit cannot be separated (conventional medicine acknowledges at least the first two; even the surgeon general of the United States has stated that mind and body are "inseparable"[79]), then we should not look only to one area for the cause and the solution. Even if the source arises in one area, the reverberations, like ripples in a pond, extend throughout the body, mind, and spirit and are soon indistinguishable as cause or effect.

To recover from bipolar disorder, we need not know the exact mechanism in operation, but we do need to address the factors that combine to produce the disorder. This means identifying and treating the imbalances in each individual case of bipolar disorder; the approach must be individualized because the combination of factors differs and the specifics of each factor vary from person to person.

With that in mind, this chapter looks at 20 factors that can play a role in bipolar disorder. While a particular factor may seem to be predominantly physical, psychological, or spiritual in nature, remember the ripple-in-the-pond effect and know that it will have an effect on the other areas as well.

20 Factors in Bipolar Disorder

The following can exacerbate or contribute to bipolar disorder:

genetic vulnerability
stress
chemical toxicity
heavy metal toxicity
food allergies
intestinal dysbiosis
sensitivity to food additives
nutritional deficiencies
    or imbalances
neurotransmitter deficiencies
    or dysfunction
hormonal imbalances
hypoglycemia
structural factors
medical conditions
medications
stimulants
lack of sleep
lack of exercise
lack of light
energy imbalances
psychospiritual issues

1. Genetic Vulnerability

"No claim of a gene for a psychiatric condition has stood the test of time, in spite of popular misinformation," states Joseph

Glenmullen, M.D., in *Prozac Backlash*.[80] This statement is made more significant when you consider the amount of research hours, energy, and money that has gone into looking for the genes.

The statistics for occurrence of mood disorders within families (see chapter 1) seem to support the existence of a genetic component. The fact that only 65 percent of the identical twins of a twin with bipolar disorder develop the disorder,[81] however, suggests that environmental factors play a role as well. This is what is meant by "genetic vulnerability"; a genetic abnormality sets the stage for environmental factors to trigger the disorder. *Environmental* in this usage simply means not genetic, so toxins, traumatic events, and nutritional deficiencies from a poor diet, for example, all fall in the environmental category.

Some kind of vulnerability is clearly operational in bipolar disorder, given the family statistics and the fact that not everyone develops the condition. The way this vulnerability is viewed depends on one's medical orientation. While conventional researchers and physicians focus exclusively on gene abnormality passed down through families as the source of the vulnerability in some people, those who understand the electromagnetic field of the human body and how energy functions in health and disease might consider the contribution of an inherited energy imbalance or an energy legacy passed down from generation to generation (see "Energy Imbalances" in this chapter).

Some scientists believe that a phenomenon called "gene penetrance" may now be operational in bipolar disorder. Gene penetrance refers to the increasing development of a genetic disorder the further along the generational chain it has been passed. In other words, descendants may be more likely than their forebears to develop bipolar disorder.[82] This phenomenon could also be viewed in energetic terms, with the energetic influence becoming more powerful the more times it is passed down, much in the way that a homeopathic remedy, which is an energy-based medicine, becomes more potent the more times it is diluted (see chapter 9).

Regardless of what genetic research discovers or how you view the inherited vulnerability, that predisposition does not translate as "hopeless or incurable," as biochemical researcher William J. Walsh, Ph.D., says in chapter 5. By considering the 19 other factors cited here and addressing those that you think or discover have relevance to your condition, you open the way for restoration of your health.

2. Stress

The subject of stress is a natural follow-up to genetic vulnerability because it is one of the major environmental influences in bipolar disorder. In fact, the rest of the factors cited in this chapter could be called stressors, in that they put stress on the system and thus add to a person's total stress load.

Chronic stress wreaks havoc on the body, mind, and spirit

Some scientists believe that a phenomenon called "gene penetrance" may now be operational in bipolar disorder. Gene penetrance refers to the increasing development of a genetic disorder the further along the generational chain it has been passed. In other words, descendants may be more likely than their forebears to develop bipolar disorder.

and creates a vicious circle. On the physical level, stress drains nutrients and lowers immunity. The nutritional deficiencies result in compromised neurochemistry in the brain, which in turn reduces the body's ability to cope with stress. Lowered immunity also reduces the stress-coping capacity and opens the body to the development of disease. In addition, it creates disturbances in the energy system of the body, which affects all levels of functioning.

Chronic stress also impairs the body's natural homeostatic ability, that is, the ability to maintain its internal balance. Someone who is born vulnerable to developing bipolar disorder already has "a diminished ability to adapt smoothly to the changing planetary environment—or to accommodate to the turmoil of chronic stress—and recover homeostatic balance once the challenges have passed," says Peter C. Whybrow, M.D., author of *A Mood Apart: The Thinker's Guide to Emotion and Its Disorders.*[83]

This means that the genetic or energetic vulnerability leaves a person less able to deal with stress.

Episodes of both depression and mania in the early course of bipolar disorder are often connected to stressful life events. As the disorder progresses, however, episodes often occur independent of life occurrences. This is known as the "kindling phenomenon," which refers to increased vulnerability to the recurrence of mood episodes, with less stress required to trigger an episode each time, until the episodes arise independent of stress and recur more and more often. Dr. Francis Mondimore calls this the point at which "the illness has become sufficiently 'kindled' that stress management no longer has much of an impact . . . "[84]

This is a strong argument for reducing the amount of stress in your life, whether through avoidance of known stressful situations, making changes in your circumstances or lifestyle, and/or practicing meditation and relaxation techniques. Attending to the rest of the factors in this chapter can significantly reduce your stress load.

3. Chemical Toxicity

Toxic overload places tremendous stress on the body and contributes to the development of disease. Humans today are exposed to an unprecedented number of chemicals. Testing of anyone on Earth, no matter how remote the area in which they live, will reveal that they are carrying at least 250 chemical contaminants in their body fat.[85] The onslaught of chemicals begins in the womb, with the transmission of toxins from the toxic mother to the fetus, and continues with breast-feeding. An infant in the United States or Europe imbibes "the maximum recommended lifetime dose of dioxin" in only six months of nursing. Dioxin, a pesticide by-product, is one of the most toxic substances on Earth.[86] The point is that we start life with an already accumulating toxic load.

In their report, *In Harm's Way—Toxic Threats to Child Development*, the Greater Boston Physicians for Social Responsibility summarize research on lead, mercury, cadmium, manganese, nicotine, pesticides (many of which are commonly used in homes and schools), and solvents used in paint, glue, and cleaning products, and dioxin and PCBs (polychlorinated biphenyls; both PCBs and dioxin stay in the food chain once they enter it, as they pervasively have).

The report notes that in one year alone (1997), industrial plants released more than a billion pounds of these chemicals directly into the environment (air, water, and land). Further, almost 75 percent of the top 20 chemicals (those released in the largest quantities) are known or suspected to be neurotoxicants.[87] (Neurotoxicants are substances that are toxic to the brain and the nervous system in general.) Other sources report that of 70,000 different chemicals being used commercially, only 10 percent have been tested for their effect on the nervous system.[88] In addition to the pesticides used directly on crops, the chemicals in the air, water, and soil are fully integrated into our food supply.

The neurotoxic effects of the chemical onslaught emerge as mood disorders, among many other symptoms and diseases. "In the earliest form of chronic toxicity, mild mood disorders predominate as the patient's chief complaint," states an official at the National Institute for Occupational Safety and Health.[89]

"Everyday chemicals have the potential to interfere with the metabolism of brain neurotransmitters or happy hormones in a myriad of pathways," says Sherry A. Rogers, M.D., author of *Depression—Cured at Last!* "They interfere with synthesis and metabolism, they block receptor sites, poison enzymes, and much more."[90]

As just one example of how this works, consider the hydrazines, a family of widely used chemicals, notably in pesticides, jet fuels, and growth retardants. Hydrazine is sprayed on potatoes to prolong their shelf life. In the body, this chemical blocks serotonin production by blocking the action of vitamin B_6, which is needed at every step in the series of enzyme actions required in the manufacture of serotonin. In just one bag of potato chips or one serving of fast-food French fries, there is sufficient hydrazine to knock out all the B_6 in your body.[91]

While we can't avoid toxic exposure entirely, given the state of our planet, avoiding the use of toxic cleaning and other home and garden products, eating organically grown food, drinking pure bottled or filtered water, and avoiding other sources of toxic exposure wherever possible can at least reduce our toxic loads.

 For information on clearing toxins from your body, home, and beyond, see Richard Leviton, *The Healthy Living Space* (Hampton Roads, 2001).

4. Heavy Metal Toxicity

As with chemicals, heavy metals contribute to the toxic burden our bodies are being forced to carry. In addition, heavy metals such as mercury, copper, lead, and aluminum have been linked to mood disorders. "Historians have theorized that one of the reasons the Roman empire declined was as a result of contamination from lead pipes," says author Catherine Carrigan. "A hundred years from now, future historians may reckon that one of the reasons depression increased so rapidly in our society was as a result of widespread exposure to toxic metals."[92]

The heavy metal mercury is well recognized as a neurotoxin, and has been for centuries. Early hatmakers contracted what was known as "mad hatter's disease," the result of poisoning from the mercury used in hatmaking, hence the saying, "mad as a hatter." Physiologically, mercury's effects on the brain arise from its ability to bond firmly with structures in the nervous system, explains Dr. Dietrich Klinghardt, whose work is featured in chapter 3.

Research shows that it is taken up in the peripheral nervous system by all nerve endings (in the tongue, lungs, intestines, and connective tissue, for example) and then transported quickly via nerves to the spinal cord and brainstem. "Once mercury has traveled up the axon, the nerve cell is impaired in its ability to detoxify itself and in its ability to nurture itself," says Dr. Klinghardt. "The cell becomes toxic and dies—or lives in a state of chronic malnutrition. . . . A multitude of illnesses, usually associated with neurological symptoms, result."[93]

Mercury is bioaccumulative, which means that it doesn't break down in the environment or in the body. The result is that it is everywhere in our environment, in our food, air, and water, and each exposure adds to our internal accumulation. Many of us also carry a source of mercury in our mouths in the form of dental fillings; so-called silver fillings are actually composed of more than 50 percent mercury. These fillings leach mercury, predominantly in the form of vapor, 80 percent of which is absorbed through the lungs into the bloodstream. Chewing raises the level of vapor emission and it remains elevated for at least 90 minutes afterward.[94]

Among the symptoms that improve after having mercury amalgam fillings replaced with nontoxic composite fillings are depression, anxiety, fatigue, lack of energy, nervousness, irritability, insomnia, headaches, memory loss, lack of concentration, allergies, gastrointestinal upset, and thyroid problems. In a survey of 762 people conducted by the Foundation for Toxic Free Dentistry of Orlando, Florida, 23.75 percent (181) of the subjects reported that they had suffered from depression prior to having their mercury fillings replaced, and 100 percent of them reported that the depression disappeared afterward.[95]

Copper is also found in dental fillings, often added as an alloy to gold fillings. Other sources of copper exposure are cigarettes, cookware, and water pipes. Lead exposure is often an occupational hazard; approximately one million Americans are exposed to lead on the job.[96] Other sources of exposure include certain glazed ceramics, old paint, water pipes, fertilizers, and soft vinyl products. In 1996, cheap vinyl miniblinds were recalled due to a high lead content. Other products with even higher lead contents are still on the market. For example, one manufacturer's rainsuit for children tested at two percent lead, which is almost one hundred times the amount allowed in miniblinds.[97]

In addition to depression, aluminum toxicity has been linked to Alzheimer's, gastrointestinal problems, and liver dysfunction.[98] Among the common sources of aluminum exposure are cookware, aluminum salts in baking powder, aluminum-containing antacids, and many antiperspirants and deodorants.

Avoiding sources of these heavy metals both reduces your overall toxic load and removes a potential source of exacerbation of your symptoms.

5. Food Allergies

Depression, fatigue, and headaches are the most common symptoms of food allergies in adults. Mood symptoms run the gamut from mild anxiety to serious depression.[99] Many people are not aware that they are suffering from food allergies, as the symptoms are often not clearly linked with ingestion of the food, as is the case when someone breaks out in a rash after eating strawberries or experiences a dangerous constriction of air passages after eating shellfish.

A discussion of allergies involves both what happens in the body on a physical level as well as the imbalance in the energy field that an allergy entails. The latter is why NAET (Nambudripad's Allergy Elimination Techniques; see chapter 8), which employs acupuncture among other techniques to restore the body's energy flow in relation to the allergen (substance to which one is sensitive or allergic), is effective in eliminating allergies. Disturbances in the flow of energy by themselves produce a range of symptoms, including mood changes.

Seeming allergies may actually be intolerances or sensitivities resulting from compromised immune and digestive systems or energy disturbances. Once these factors are eliminated or eased, the food intolerances may disappear.

Food intolerances occur when the body doesn't digest food adequately, which results in large undigested protein molecules entering the intestines from the stomach. When poor digestion is chronic, these large molecules push through the lining of the intestines, creating the condition known as leaky gut, and enter the bloodstream. There, these substances are out of context, not recognized as food molecules, and so are regarded as foreign invaders.

The immune system sends an antibody (also called an immunoglobulin) to bind with the foreign protein (antigen), a process which produces the chemicals of allergic response. The antigen-antibody combination is known as a circulating immune complex, or CIC. Normally, a CIC is destroyed or removed from the body, but under conditions of weakened immunity, CICs tend to accumulate in the blood, putting the body on allergic alert, if you will. Thereafter, whenever the person eats the food in question, an allergic reaction follows.

It is important to consider here the concept of "brain allergies." Until recently, allergies were thought to affect only the mucous membranes, the respiratory tract, and the skin. A growing body of evidence indicates that an allergy can have profound effects on the brain and, as a result, on behavior. An allergy or intolerance that affects the brain is known as a brain allergy or a cerebral allergy.

Gluten (a protein found in wheat and other grains) intolerance is especially indicated in bipolar disorder. See chapter 6 for a full discussion of this.

The intestinal dysfunction inherent in food allergies contributes to mood states, as discussed in the following section.

6. Intestinal Dysbiosis

Intestinal dysbiosis means an imbalance of the flora that normally inhabit the intestines. Among these flora are the beneficial bacteria (known as probiotics) *Lactobacillus acidophilus* and *Bifidobacterium bifidum,* potentially harmful bacteria such as *E. coli* and *Clostridium,* and the fungus *Candida albicans.* When the balance among these flora is disturbed, the microorganisms held in check by the beneficial bacteria proliferate and release toxins that compromise intestinal function. This has far-reaching effects in the body and on the mind.

Research has revealed that what passes through the lining of the intestines (see "Food Allergies") can make its way through the bloodstream to the brain.[100] As an example of just one of the results of this relationship, in the brain certain intestinal bacteria can interfere with neurotransmitter function.[101] Depression and fatigue are two of the many health problems that can result from intestinal dysbiosis.

Dysbiosis contributes to a buildup of toxins in the body in two ways. One, the harmful bacteria's normal metabolism processes release toxic by-products. Two, a compromised intestinal system cannot adequately filter toxins, which is one of the important functions of the intestinal lining. Normally, bile from the liver goes through the intestines where toxins are filtered out, and the bile is then recirculated, cleansed. When the intestines are not working correctly, bile is returned to the body with the old toxicity. This condition is known as enterohepatic toxicity (*entero* for intestines and *hepatic* for liver).

Depression, fatigue, and headaches, among numerous other symptoms, can result from an intestinal overgrowth of *Candida albicans,* the yeast-like fungus normally found in the body. Mercury is often implicated in this overgrowth because "the purpose of *Candida* in the human being is to protect the body from mercury by absorbing it," says Thomas M. Rau, M.D., director of the Paracelsus Klinik in Lustmühle, Switzerland. The mechanism was never intended, however, to deal with large amounts of mercury. Nevertheless, when mercury levels in the body are high, the population of *Candida* multiplies in a vain attempt to deal with the heavy metal load.

Through its normal metabolic processes, *Candida* releases substances that are toxic to the brain and interfere with neurotransmitter activity.[102] Another mechanism by which *Candida* overgrowth has an impact on mood is that the intestinal lining becomes inflamed, which interferes with the absorption of nutrients.[103] As discussed later, nutritional deficiencies are implicated in bipolar disorder.

Candida overgrowth occurs when something intervenes to disturb the normal balance of flora in the intestinal environment. The main culprit in throwing off the balance is antibiotics, particularly the repeated use of antibiotics, which kill all the beneficial bacteria that keep potentially harmful flora such as *Candida* in check. Weakened immunity may also be a factor in yeast overgrowth.

Eliminating foods that "feed" *Candida* is a common treatment approach to restoring intestinal balance. The so-called *Candida* diet emphasizes avoiding all forms and sources of sugar, including fruit and fruit juice, carbohydrates, and fermented yeast products. According to Dr. Rau, however, the relationship between mercury and *Candida* means that until you detoxify the body of the mercury, you won't be able to get rid of the *Candida* overgrowth on any lasting basis, no matter how perfect your diet or what antifungal drug or natural substance you take. The fungus will just keep coming back.[104]

In addition to antibiotics, anti-inflammatory drugs, food allergies, and a poor diet can all help create intestinal dysbiosis.

7. Sensitivity to Food Additives

Food additives can produce a range of effects from depression, insomnia, nervousness, and hyperactivity to dizziness, blurred vision, and migraines. Research has established that aspartame (an artificial sweetener), aspartic acid (an amino acid in aspartame), glutamic acid (found in flavor enhancers and salt substitutes), and the artificial flavoring MSG (monosodium glutamate) are neurotoxins.[105] Aspartame and MSG are particularly implicated in depression. Depression is one of the frequent complaints to the FDA (Food and Drug Administration) associated with ingestion of aspartame.[106] Aspartame alters amino acid ratios and blocks serotonin production.[107] MSG has been shown to affect serotonin levels.[108]

The more than 3,000 additives used in commercially prepared food have not been tested by their manufacturers for their effects on the nervous system or on behavior.[109] In addition to those mentioned, common food additives are artificial flavoring, artificial preservatives (BHA, BHT, and TBHQ are in this category), artificial coloring/food dyes, thickeners, moisteners, and artificial sweeteners.

Sensitivity to food additives varies; a high sensitivity may reflect an already large toxic load or weakened immunity. Noticing if your symptoms worsen after ingesting certain foods can start the process of elimination for determining which additives, if any, are problematic for you.

8. Nutritional Deficiencies and Imbalances

Nutritional deficiencies and imbalances are a common feature in bipolar disorder and other "mental" illnesses. Correcting these often produces dramatic improvement. Unfortunately, nutrient status testing and intervention are not standard practice in conventional psychiatric medicine.

"Nutrient-related disorders are always treatable and deficiencies are usually curable. To ignore their existence is tantamount to malpractice," states Richard A. Kunin, M.D.,[110] a practitioner of orthomolecular medicine (the supplemental use of substances that occur naturally in the body, such as vitamins, minerals, amino acids, and enzymes, to maintain health and treat disease).

Nutrient deficiencies most implicated in bipolar disorder are essential fatty acids, amino acids, the B vitamins, magnesium, and zinc.

Again, no two people with bipolar disorder will have the exact same nutritional condition. Blood chemistry analysis can determine the precise status of your nutrient levels. With this information, therapeutic intervention can then be tailored to your specific nutrient needs. Random supplementation may not address those needs and may even contribute to further skewing of nutrient ratios.

While other factors such as absorption problems or even a genetic disorder may be involved in nutritional deficiencies and imbalances, poor diet is a primary cause. Any factor that contributes to your vulnerability should be avoided if you suffer from bipolar disorder. Erratic eating habits or a nutrient-depleted diet, as in junk-food, fast-food, processed-food diets, definitely fall into the category of contributing to vulnerability. Without the proper nutrients to feed your brain and nervous system, you are more likely to cycle in and out of depression and mania.

Essential Fatty Acids: Research has discovered a link between lipids and mental disorders. Lipids are fats or oils, which are comprised of fatty acids. Examples of saturated fatty acids are animal fats and other fats, such as coconut oil, that are solid at room temperature. Examples of unsaturated fatty acids, which remain liquid at room temperature, are certain plant and fish oils. Essential fatty acids (EFAs) are unsaturated fats required for many metabolic actions in the body.

There are two main types of EFAs: omega-3 and omega-6. The primary omega-3 EFAs are ALA (alpha-linolenic acid), DHA (docosahexaenoic acid), and EPA (eicosapentaenoic acid). ALA is found in flaxseed and canola oils, pumpkins, walnuts, and soybeans, while DHA and EPA are found in the oils of cold-water fish such as salmon, cod, and mackerel.

Two important types of omega-6 EFAs are GLA (gamma-linolenic acid) and linoleic acid or cis-linoleic acid. Evening primrose, black currant, and borage oils are sources of GLA, while linoleic acid is found in most plants and vegetable oils, notably safflower, corn, peanut, and sesame oils. The body converts omega-3 and omega-6 EFAs into prostaglandins, which are hormone-like substances involved in many metabolic functions, including inflammatory processes.

The ratio of omega-3 to omega 6-EFAs is skewed in the standard American diet, which is deficient in omega 3s. High consumption of hydrogenated oils and beef contributes to the skewed ratio. Hydrogenated oils (which are oils processed to extend shelf life) are detrimental in two ways: not only does refining oil reduce its omega-3 content, but hydrogenated oils also take up the fatty acid receptor sites and interfere with normal fatty acid metabolism. Hydrogenated oils, also known as trans-fatty acids, are found in margarine, commercial baked goods, crackers, cookies, and other products. The problem with conventionally raised beef cattle is that they are grain-fed rather than grass-fed; grain is high in omega 6 and low in omega 3, while grass provides a more balanced ratio.[111]

Andrew Stoll, M.D., a psychopharmacology researcher and an assistant professor of psychiatry at Harvard Medical School, states: "Omega-3 fatty acids . . . are essential nutrients for human brain development and general health. Over the past 50 to 100 years, there has been an accelerated deficiency of omega-3 fatty acids in most Western countries. There is emerging evidence that this progressive omega-3 deficiency is responsible, at least in part, for the rise in the incidence of heart disease, asthma, bipolar disorder, major depression, and perhaps autism."[112] (Note that in certain cases of bipolar disorder, those involving a condition called pyroluria, the EFA that is deficient is omega-6; see chapter 5.)

> **Nerve cells in the brain contain high levels of omega-3 fatty acids. A deficiency could obviously have serious consequences. There is a large body of research demonstrating links between essential fatty acids and bipolar disorder, depression, and other mental disorders.**

Lipids are necessary for the health of the blood vessels that feed the brain and comprise 50 to 60 percent of the brain's solid matter.[113] More specifically, nerve cells in the brain contain high levels of omega-3 fatty acids.[114] A deficiency could obviously have serious consequences. There is a large body of research demonstrating links between essential fatty acids and bipolar disorder, depression, and other mental disorders. The following is just a sampling of the extensive research findings:

- In one placebo-controlled double-blind study by Dr. Stoll, 64 percent of subjects given omega-3 fatty acid supplements (fish oil) experienced improvement in their manic-depressive symptoms, compared to only 18 percent of those taking a placebo.[115]

- There is a correlation between severity of depression and omega-3 fatty acid levels. The lower the levels the more severe the depression.[116]

- Low DHA levels have been linked to low brain serotonin levels, which are associated with a greater tendency toward depression, suicide, and violence.[117]

- Research has found that EPA can be at least as effective as antipsychotics (often given to those with bipolar disorder), and in some cases EPA supplementation can obviate medication.[118]

- Low-fat diets, which typically involve a reduced intake of omega-3 and an increased intake of omega-6 EFAs, can increase the risk of depression.[119]

- One study correlated fish consumption and the incidence of major depression per 100 people in nine countries. The countries with the lowest consumption of fish had the highest incidence of depression, and vice versa.[120]

 For more about essential fatty acid supplementation in the treatment of bipolar disorder, see chapters 3, 4, 5, and 6.

Amino Acids: The production of neurotransmitters that regulate mood requires the presence of certain amino acids or precursors. Tryptophan is the amino acid precursor for serotonin; phenylalanine and tyrosine are the precursors for dopamine and norepinephrine. (GABA is an amino acid that also acts as a neurotransmitter.)

Amino acids are the basic building blocks for neurotransmitters, enzymes, hormones, and other proteins. The body does not manufacture most of the amino acids it requires, so they must be obtained through protein in the diet. With a deficient diet, the body is not able to produce sufficient neurotransmitters, which can contribute to bipolar disorder and depression, among other conditions.

Amino acid supplementation can be effective in alleviating bipolar disorder and serves as a safe and far less expensive alternative to prescription drugs that target the neurotransmitters. Although it may not address the root cause of amino acid deficiency, such as a poor diet, it corrects the problem, unlike antidepressants and other drugs. It also increases the supply of neurotransmitters naturally, by simply supplying the body with the building materials it needs, instead of forcing the brain and the neurotransmitters into unnatural function to keep the neuro-transmitters available.

Research has found tryptophan may be beneficial in the treatment of mania, depression, anxiety, panic disorder, sleep disorders, and psychosis.[121] One study of the effects of tryptophan supplementation was conducted with 11 patients whose depression was so severe that they were hospitalized. After just a month of supplementation, standard psychiatric tests revealed that the overall depressive states of the 11 patients had dropped by 38 percent. In seven of the 11, guilt, anxiety, weight loss, and insomnia were significantly reduced.[122]

In the body, tryptophan is converted into 5-HTP (5-hydroxy tryptophan) and then into serotonin. A plant extract form of 5-HTP, available as a supplement, can also be used to boost serotonin levels. A Swiss study found that the antidepressant effects of 5-HTP were equal to those of the conventional SSRI Luvox (fluvoxamine), with fewer of the subjects in the 5-HTP group experiencing side effects. (High dosages of 5-HTP may produce nausea, other gastrointestinal distress, and drowsiness.)

Research on phenylalanine and tyrosine indicates that they can also be beneficial in the treatment of depression.[123]

GABA has proven useful in the treatment of mania, acute agitation, anxiety, nervous tension, hyperactivity, insomnia, and other brain and nervous disorders. One of the signs of GABA deficiency is excessive mental activity, as is characteristic in a manic episode.[124]

For a full discussion of amino acids and their use in bipolar disorder, see chapter 6.

Vitamins and Minerals: As you can see from the list of effects from vitamin deficiency in the accompanying sidebar, the whole vitamin B family is essential for mental health. As with amino acids, B vitamins are found in protein foods. Someone with an amino acid deficiency is often deficient in B vitamins as well. Based on the clinical experience of the practitioners in this book, the most common vitamin deficiencies associated with bipolar disorder are vitamin B_3 (niacin/niacinamide), vitamin B_6 (pyridoxine), B_{12} (cobalamin), and folic acid (a member of the vitamin

Mood-Related Effects of Vitamin Deficiencies

The following are the results of deficiencies in vitamin C and the B complex vitamin family that relate to the symptoms of mood disorder.

Deficient Vitamin	Resulting Behavior
Ascorbic acid (vitamin C)	Depression, hysteria, confusion, lassitude, hypochondriasis
Biotin	Depression, extreme lassitude, somnolence
Folic acid	Depression, apathy, insomnia, irritability, forgetfulness, delirium, dementia, psychosis
Vitamin B_1 (thiamin)	Depression, apathy, anxiety, irritability, memory loss, personality changes, emotional instability
Vitamin B_2 (riboflavin)	Depression, insomnia, mental sluggishness
Vitamin B_3 (niacin/niacinamide)	Depression, mania, anxiety, apathy, hyperirritability, emotional instability, memory and concentration problems
Vitamin B_5 (pantothenic acid)	Depression, restlessness, irritability, fatigue, quarrelsomeness
Vitamin B_6 (pyridoxine)	Depression, irritability, nervousness, insomnia, poor dream recall
Vitamin B_{12} (cobalamin)	Depression, mood swings, irritability, confusion, memory loss, hallucinations, delusions, paranoia, psychotic states

Source: Reprinted by permission of Rita Elkins, from her book *Depression and Natural Medicine: A Nutritional Approach to Depression and Mood Swings* (Pleasant Grove, Utah: Woodland Publishing, 1995): 75.

B family), all of which are vital to neurotransmitter function. Biochemical researcher William Walsh, Ph.D., has found that a genetic disorder, which causes severe deficiency in both vitamin B_6 and zinc, can be a factor in bipolar disorder (see chapter 5).

Inositol (another member of the B complex family), phosphatidyl choline (found in lecithin), and magnesium are important for nervous system balance as well. Phosphatidyl choline exerts benefits for mania, while inositol does the same for depressive episodes.[125] Magnesium, which functions in ratio to calcium, may be of use in bipolar disorder for the same reason that calcium channel blockers are sometimes prescribed, for the calming effect that results from blocking calcium channels in cells.[126] Supplementation with magnesium can help restore the proper ratio and action of the two minerals. In addition, magnesium enhances vitamin B_6 activity and, taken as a supplement, helps prevent the magnesium deficiency that can result from high doses of B_6.

Poor diet and malabsorption due to gastrointestinal dysfunction are common causes of nutritional deficiencies. The depleted mineral content of the soil in which crops are grown, which translates into food with a lower mineral content than our forebears enjoyed, is a factor as well. Finally, many lifestyle practices and attributes of modern life deplete us of vitamins and minerals, regardless of how well we eat: stress, smoking, alcohol, caffeine, pollution, heavy metals such as the mercury in our dental fillings.

Given these factors, the recommended daily allowance (RDA: purportedly, the amount of individual vitamins and minerals our body requires daily, whether from food or supplements) is likely far below our nutritive needs, in most cases. The RDA standard is based on a group norm for preventing nutritional deficiencies. There are two problems with that. One, individual needs diverge widely and two, the level of deficiency the RDAs are designed to avoid is severe. The systems of the body can begin to be compromised long before that degree of deficiency registers. In other words, if you use the RDAs as your guideline, you could be walking around with moderate nutritional deficiencies.

Increasing your intake of foods that contain the nutrients cited above is a good idea if you are deficient. The following are dietary sources of these nutrients:

- Folic acid: brewer's yeast, green leafy vegetables, wheat germ, soybeans, legumes, asparagus, broccoli, oranges, sunflower seeds

- Inositol: citrus, nuts, seeds, legumes

- Magnesium: parsnips, tofu, buckwheat, beans, leafy green vegetables, wheat germ, blackstrap molasses, kelp, brewer's yeast, nuts, seeds, bananas, avocado, dairy, seafood

- Vitamin B_3: brewer's yeast, rice bran, peanuts, eggs, milk, fish, legumes, avocado, liver and other organ meats

- Vitamin B_6: brewer's yeast, wheat germ, bananas, seeds, nuts, legumes, avocado, leafy green vegetables, potatoes, cauliflower, chicken, whole grains

- Vitamin B_{12}: liver, kidneys, eggs, clams, oysters, fish, dairy

- Zinc: oysters, herring, sunflower seeds, pumpkin seeds, lima beans, legumes, soybeans, wheat germ, brewer's yeast, dairy.

9. Neurotransmitter Deficiencies or Dysfunction

The role of the neurotransmitters serotonin, dopamine, norepinephrine, and GABA in bipolar disorder is covered in chapter 1. While the theory that problems with these brain chemicals is behind bipolar disorder has not been proven, the clinical results of supporting neurotransmitters with their amino acid precursors and other nutrients indicates involvement, if not causality.

The problem with the neurotransmitters can be one of supply, function, or both. A normal level of a given neurotransmitter does not guarantee that the mind and body will receive its benefits. For example, despite high blood levels of the neurotransmitter serotonin, reduced uptake in the brain may mean that the availability of this vital nerve messenger is actually limited.[127]

Attempting to correct neurotransmitter supply or even function does not address the root problem of why the supply is low or the neurotransmitters are not working properly. As you will learn in part II of this book, treating the root problems, which range from the physical to the spiritual, often results in the neurotransmitter deficiency or dysfunction self-correcting as the body is restored to its innate ability to heal itself.

10. Hormonal Imbalances

Hormones "are probably second only to the chemicals of the brain in shaping how we feel and behave."[128] Hormonal imbalances influence brain chemistry and the nervous system.[129] "Neurons are very sensitive to rapid changes in their hormonal environment," states Dr. Whybrow. "Any rapid change in these hormone levels . . . demands immediate accommodation, and while adaptation is proceeding, mood is commonly unstable."[130] The hormones particularly implicated in mood are thyroid hormones, adrenal hormones (cortisol, DHEA, epinephrine, and norepinephrine), and reproductive hormones (estrogen, progesterone, and testosterone).[131]

The symptoms of thyroid and adrenal gland diseases are similar to those of depressive and manic episodes.[132] Hypo- and hyperthyroidism (an underactive and overactive thyroid, respectively) are two thyroid conditions that can masquerade as bipolar disorder. Hypothyroidism is often overlooked as a cause because it can be at a subclinical level and still produce mood symptoms. This can become a vicious circle, as taking lithium can cause hypothyroidism.[133]

Of the adrenal hormones, too little DHEA (dehydroepiandrosterone) or too high levels of the stress hormone cortisol have been linked with depression.[134] As discussed in the previous chapter, epinephrine, or adrenaline, is involved in the stress response and anxiety, while norepinephrine, the form of adrenaline found in the brain, is one of the "feel good" neuro-transmitters and as such has influence in affective disorders. Chronic stress, which involves continual release of the adrenal stress hormones, compromises the body's adaptive capacity, leaving a person with bipolar disorder more vulnerable. Even a small stressor can then trigger a manic or depressive episode.[135]

In women, too little of the hormone estrogen in relation to the other reproductive hormones tends to produce depression, while too much estrogen in relation to other hormones tends to result in anxiety.[136] Too little progesterone can also lead to depression; this is often the problem with both premenstrual and postpartum depression.[137] Testosterone deficiency in both men and women (yes, women have testosterone) can result in depression as well.[138]

Postpartum mania due to the hormonal changes following childbirth can occur in women who do not have bipolar disorder, but women who do have it, or who have a family history of it, are 20 to 30 times more likely to have a manic episode triggered by childbirth.[139]

Toxic exposure, stress, diet, and exercise can all affect hormonal levels and balance.

11. Hypoglycemia

Hypoglycemia is a condition in which the glucose level in the blood is low, and is otherwise known as low blood sugar. The symptoms are restlessness, irritability, fatigue, and, when severe, mental disturbances.

Psychiatrist and orthomolecular physician Michael Lesser, M.D., among others, observed in clinical practice that patients with bipolar disorder also have "widely swinging blood sugar curves." In charting a patient's moods in relation to blood sugar levels, Dr. Lesser discovered that the patient's depressions corresponded to times of low blood sugar. "Lithium, the mineral which 'curbs' the wide oscillations in mood characteristic of manic-depressive illness, also levels out the oscillations in blood sugar levels of manic-depressives," he says. "Perhaps this is one of the reasons it works."[140]

Of hypoglycemia in mood disorders, Dr. Walsh (see chapter 5) says, "This problem doesn't appear to be the cause . . . but instead is an aggravating factor which can trigger striking symptoms."[141]

12. Structural Factors

Structural factors such as cranial compression can be a component in bipolar disorder. Such compression, which is the result of skull distortion, can occur through birth trauma or a later physical trauma, such as a car accident. The impact of cranial compression has far-reaching effects throughout the body, but in the head the compression exerts pressure on the brain and cranial nerves, which compromises neurotransmitter function and brain function in general. This factor is explored in depth in chapter 7.

13. Medical Conditions

According to the *DSM-IV*, the following medical conditions can produce mood symptoms that can be mistaken for bipolar disorder: Parkinson's disease; Huntington's disease; cerebrovascular disease, including stroke, hyper- and hypothyroidism (see "Hormonal Problems"); lupus; viral infections, including HIV, hepatitis, and mononucleosis; and pancreatic cancer. The *DSM-IV* also cites vitamin B_{12} deficiency as a medical condition that can cause mood disorder.[142]

Researchers have long been exploring a possible connection between viruses and bipolar disorder. While a viral cause has not been identified, prenatal viral infections may be implicated, as there is evidence that people who suffer from bipolar disorder are more often born during winter months.[143]

14. Medications/Drugs

"Probably all antidepressants and stimulants are capable of causing mania," state Drs. Breggin and Cohen. Along with those two categories of drugs, the *DSM-IV* cites the following as sources of drug-induced mood symptoms: analgesics (pain relievers), anesthetics, anticonvulsants, antihypertensives (for high blood pressure), antipsychotics, antiulcer medications, benzodiazepines (tranquilizers), heart medications, oral contraceptives, muscle relaxants, and steroids, among others.[144] Other medications that can cause depression are antihistamines, anti-inflammatories, drugs that lower cholesterol, and quinolone antibiotics (Cipro and Floxin).[145]

A bipolar episode can also be triggered when a person stops taking a psychiatric medication. Lithium, major tranquilizers, and antidepressants can all produce this effect. A shorter time to recurrence of an episode is also associated with abruptly reducing the dosage of these drugs.[146] Research also indicates that at least for some people the very drugs they take to treat their psychiatric condition can in reality worsen the progression of that condition, making it a necessity after more than three years of usage to stay on the drugs.[147]

Patty Duke believes that anesthesia and cortisone (a steroid) were responsible for triggering two of her episodes. The first manic episode she can recall came when she was 18 and had emergency surgery for a ruptured appendix and an ovarian cyst. "[A]fter I came home from the hospital, I literally went crazy. I was hallucinating and raving and ranting and not sleeping and not eating and spending a lot of money. . . . I recovered from this manic episode, which I'm convinced was brought on by the anesthesia I had during the surgery."[148] Many years later, another episode (with this one, she was at last diagnosed with manic-depression) followed a cortisone shot. Duke was seeing a psychiatrist at the time. "He told me that he had suspected for a long time that I might have this condition," she recalls, "and he believed that it was the shot of cortisone that had triggered this episode."[149]

15. Stimulants and Alcohol

Caffeine, cocaine, and amphetamines are well known as substances to avoid (or in the case of caffeine, limit) if you have bipolar disorder. Research has found that the level of caffeine ingested is positively correlated with the degree of mental illness among psychiatric patients,[150] meaning that the more caffeine taken in, the worse the symptoms. People who drink a lot of coffee test higher for anxiety and depression and are also more likely than their more abstemious counterparts to develop psychotic disorders.[151] Some people give up or cut down on coffee and black tea, but forget about the high caffeine content in colas. It is not unusual to hear people with bipolar disorder say that they were living on cigarettes and Pepsi or Coke before a manic episode started.

Caffeine does a lot more than give you a jittery edge. It actually affects your neurotransmitters, stimulating the release of nor-epinephrine and others. Habitual excessive intake can leave you with a neurotransmitter deficit, along with hypoglycemia, and nutritional deficiencies, as it interferes with the absorption of important nutrients such as B vitamins, magnesium, calcium, potassium, and zinc.[152] Note the overlap with nutritional deficiencies often present in bipolar disorder.

Obviously, for someone prone to mania, taking stimulants is a risky choice. The *DSM-IV* cites both use of, and withdrawal from, cocaine and amphetamines as able to produce mood disorders. Dr. Whybrow notes that "in individuals of bipolar temperament, cocaine commonly will precipitate a sustained manic episode . . . "[153]

Alcohol also interferes with normal neurotransmitter function, by impeding the supply of tryptophan to the brain and thus reducing serotonin formation. This can cause depression and insomnia. As with caffeine, habitual drinking of alcoholic beverages is associated with hypoglycemia and nutritional deficiencies, notably of B vitamins, vitamin C, folic acid, zinc, potassium, and magnesium.[154]

16. Lack of Sleep

There is a strong connection between sleep deprivation and the onset of a manic episode. Even one night without sleep can be problematic for those who suffer from bipolar disorder. Long-distance jet travel, pulling an "all-nighter" in cramming for exams, and medical or family emergencies that result in sleep deprivation have all been associated with manic onset.[155]

Sleep deprivation can trigger a depressive episode as well, or cause a switch from one pole to the other. A National Institute of Mental Health study found that following just one night without sleep, a group of people with rapid-cycling bipolar disorder

who were in a depressive episode experienced a switch into mania or hypomania the very next day.[156]

17. Lack of Exercise

Exercise stimulates the release of mood-regulating epinephrine, norepinephrine, and serotonin, along with endorphins, chemicals that lift our mood and reduce our stress level. Exercise can alleviate depression, anxiety, hyperactivity, irritability, insomnia, and schizophrenic symptoms.[158] A German study of people with major depression found that exercise (30 minutes of walking daily) reduced their depression in less than the time it typically takes antidepressants to work. Another study of depression in older adults found that exercise was more effective than antidepressants in alleviating the mood disorder.[159] Research has also demonstrated that jogging for half an hour three times weekly can be equally or more beneficial for mental health than psychotherapy.[160]

Exercise increases oxygen supply to the brain, which improves cerebral function and the ability to cope with stress.[161] Exercise also helps flush toxins out of the body, which as discussed previously has beneficial effects on mood and overall health.

18. Lack of Light

A deficiency in exposure to full-spectrum light (sunlight or indoor lighting that employs full-spectrum light bulbs) is linked to emotional instability, hyperactivity, anxiety, irritability, reduced ability to cope with stress, fatigue, apathy, seasonal affective disorder (SAD) and other types of depression, nutrient absorption problems, glandular problems, and weakened immunity, among other symptoms and conditions.[162]

For many people, lack of light has become a daily, round-the-year reality as a result of our technological age, which has so many of us spending the vast majority of our time indoors under artificial (non-full-spectrum) light.

The relationship of mood to light is reflected in the fact that bipolar disorder can have a seasonal pattern, with depressive episodes typically occurring in the seasons when there is reduced light—fall or winter. Manic episodes occur most frequently in the late summer. . . . Spending more time outdoors and using full-spectrum light bulbs in your indoor environments are steps you can take to ameliorate lack of light.

Lack of light results in lower levels of serotonin. It also contributes to sleep disorders such as insomnia because it interferes with melatonin function. Melatonin, a hormone important in sleep regulation, is manufactured from serotonin. This helps to explain the intimate relationship between depression and sleep problems. The pineal gland, which manufactures melatonin, depends upon the proper cycle of darkness and light to stimulate or inhibit production. The body runs on a 24-hour cycle known as a circadian rhythm. The brain sets the body's internal clock to observe this cycle. People with bipolar disorder are particularly affected by any disruption of their internal clock. As their adaptive mechanisms are compromised, mood disturbances may follow.[163]

The relationship of mood to light is reflected in the fact that bipolar disorder can have a seasonal pattern, with depressive episodes typically occurring in the seasons when there is reduced light—fall or winter. Manic episodes occur most frequently in the late summer. Suicides happen most often in the spring and fall, when the relationship of light and dark is undergoing the fastest changes.[164]

Spending more time outdoors and using full-spectrum light bulbs in your indoor environments are steps you can take to ameliorate lack of light. For a more focused treatment, light box therapy, in which you are exposed to more intensive full-spectrum light, may help.

19. Energy Imbalances

There are a number of different ways to discuss the flow of energy in the human body. Physiologically, the salient point for mood disorders is that the nervous system operates on electrical charges. Extending outward, you could speak of the body's electromagnetic field and the far-reaching effects on mood and health caused by disturbances in that field (see chapter 3).

If you regard energy from the perspective of traditional Chinese medicine (which includes acupuncture), you analyze disturbance in the individual's vital force, or *qi,* as manifested by disturbed energy flow along the meridians, or energy channels, throughout the body (see chapter 8). If you consider energy from a shamanic or psychic viewpoint, you might explore the presence of foreign energy in an individual's energy field (see chapter 10). Homeopathy is also an energy-based medicine, whose remedies work to resolve a condition by restoring a person's energy to its natural equilibrium, which restores balance to the body, mind, and spirit (see chapter 9).

Whatever language you choose to employ to describe the phenomenon, a disturbance in an individual's energy field can contribute to mood disorders. The relationship of energy to other factors can be cyclical, with physical factors (such as nutritional deficiencies) or psychological or spiritual issues causing or being caused by a disturbance in energy flow. As mentioned in the earlier section on genetic factors, an inherited energy imbalance or an energy legacy passed down from generation to generation may also be operational (see chapter 3).

In Their Own Words

"Chemistry isn't everything. Focusing only on chemistry is mindless, but focusing solely on psychosocial influences is brainless."[165]

—Robert Boorstin, diagnosed with bipolar disorder at 24

"I don't believe anyone with manic depression can truly benefit from talk therapy until the chemical imbalance is fixed."[166]

—Patty Duke

More detailed discussions of energy and methods for removing energy disturbances can be found throughout part II.

20. Psychospiritual Issues

As noted, psychological/ emotional and spiritual issues have the capacity to throw the energy system out of balance and vice versa. Along with their effect on mood and emotional stability, mind and spirit issues can produce a myriad of physical effects throughout the body, which in turn can compound bipolar disorder.

In keeping with the knowledge of the inseparability of body, mind, and spirit, it is important to consider possible issues in each as contributing to your bipolar disorder. Psychotherapy is one avenue for exploring the psychological and spiritual dimensions. Aside from the causal contributions in these areas, psychotherapy can provide an important forum for processing all the issues that arise from being diagnosed with, and living with, bipolar disorder. It could be considered as psychological and spiritual housecleaning or the maintenance work that taking good care of something requires. Taking good care of yourself means attending to the needs of body, mind, and spirit.

Many people with bipolar disorder find psychotherapy a vital part of their treatment program. As one person with bipolar disorder states it, "[P]sychotherapy heals, it makes some sense of the confusion, it reins in the terrifying thoughts and feelings, it brings back hope, and the possibility of learning from it all."[167]

A short-term intervention called cognitive therapy has been helpful to some people. Cognitive therapy operates on the principle that thoughts determine moods and emotions. While this is not to say that people with bipolar disorder ought to be able to control their mood swings, the therapy has application for learning how to monitor one's thinking as a warning of the early stages of an episode. Forewarned, people can then consciously change the thinking they have learned to recognize as their characteristically depressive or manic thinking, get more sleep, eat better, make sure they are exercising, or take other measures that they have learned can help them avert an episode. As one man who found cognitive therapy useful says, "I monitor my thinking patterns as an index of my emotional balance—rather like checking the blood sugar level in diabetes."[168]

Bipolar disorder is a complex condition. No single factor is responsible for creating it, and no single therapeutic measure can reverse it. This means that you must discover what factors are involved in your case and take steps to ameliorate them.

The contribution of body, mind, and spirit elements in bipolar disorder is fully explored in part II. The first chapter provides a model that will help you make sense of the various levels of healing and how they relate to each other.

Action Plan

As a summary of the information in this chapter, the following are steps you can take to eliminate the causes, triggers, and contributors to your bipolar disorder.

• Find ways to reduce or manage the stress in your life. Meditation and relaxation techniques can be beneficial.

• Reduce your toxic exposure wherever possible. Avoid using toxic house and garden products; eat organically grown food; and drink pure water instead of tap water.

• Reduce your heavy metal exposure by avoiding sources of copper, lead, aluminum, and mercury wherever possible. You may want to investigate having your mercury dental fillings replaced with nonmercury amalgams; hair analysis and other tests can determine if the level of mercury in your body is high.

- Avoid foods and other substances to which you are allergic, or get allergy treatment such as NAET to eliminate the problem (see chapter 8). If you suspect you have allergies, but don't know to what, NAET can help you identify allergens. Determine if you have a gluten intolerance (see chapter 6).

- Address any intestinal or digestive dysfunction, such as an overgrowth of *Candida.* Taking probiotics helps improve digestion.

- Avoid food additives, particularly if your symptoms seem to worsen after ingesting additives.

- Eat a healthful, balanced diet. Avoid junk food, fast food, and processed food.

- Have your biochemical status checked to identify any nutritional deficiencies or imbalances, and take the appropriate supplements to correct them (see chapters 4 and 5).

- Deficiencies or imbalances in essential fatty acids and amino acids can contribute to neurotransmitter dysfunction. Consider whether you are a candidate for supplementation (see chapters 3–6).

- Have your doctor check for hormonal imbalances.

- Consult with your doctor about hypoglycemia. If you have this condition, there are dietary practices you can follow to correct it.

- Consider consulting a cranial osteopath to eliminate structural factors that may be contributing to your bipolar disorder (see chapter 7). Cranial compression can interfere with nervous system function.

- Work with your doctor to determine if you have any medical conditions that produce bipolar symptoms.

- Consult your doctor about whether any medications you are taking might be contributing to your bipolar disorder. Also ask about any antidepressants you are taking or considering taking; some can produce mania.

- Limit or avoid intake of alcohol and caffeine. Avoid recreational drugs, especially stimulants such as cocaine and amphetamines.

- Get sufficient sleep. Try to avoid "all-nighters."

- Get regular exercise.

- Make sure to spend time outdoors every day. If lack of light is a problem for you, consider using full-spectrum light bulbs in your house or getting light therapy.

- Address energy imbalances through acupuncture, homeopathy, and other forms of energy medicine (see chapters 3 and 8–10).

- Explore psychospiritual issues through psychotherapy or other modalities (see chapters 3 and 10).

PART II

Natural Medicine Treatments for Bipolar Disorder

3 A Model for Healing

While many people speak generally of the body-mind-spirit connection, Dietrich Klinghardt, M.D., Ph.D., based in Bellevue, Washington, has developed a detailed paradigm that explains that connection in terms of Five Levels of Healing: the Physical Level, the Electromagnetic Level, the Mental Level, the Intuitive Level, and the Spiritual Level.

Dr. Klinghardt is internationally acclaimed for this brilliant and comprehensive model of healing, for his expertise in neural therapy, and for several effective therapeutic techniques he has developed (see "About the Therapies and Techniques" at the end of this chapter). He trains doctors around the world in his model and techniques and is perhaps the person most responsible for bringing neural therapy to the attention of the medical and lay communities.

The Five Levels of Healing model provides a comprehensive way to approach and understand many chronic illnesses, including bipolar disorder. Health and illness are a reflection of the state of these five levels. Bipolar disorder, like any health problem, can originate on any of the five levels. A basic principle of Dr. Klinghardt's paradigm is that an interference or imbalance on one level, if untreated, spreads upward or downward to the other levels. Thus bipolar disorder can involve multiple levels, sometimes even all five, if the originating imbalance was not correctly addressed.

Another basic principle is that healing interventions can be implemented at any of the levels. Unless upper-level imbalances are addressed, restoring balance at the lower levels will not produce long-lasting effects. This provides an answer to why rebalancing the biochemistry of the brain does not resolve some cases of bipolar disorder. Treating the chemistry only addresses the Physical Level of illness and healing and leaves the causes at the Intuitive Level, for example, intact. The brain chemistry will soon be thrown off again by the downward cascade of this imbalance.

The Five Levels of Healing model also provides a useful framework for the natural medicine therapies covered in the rest of this book. You will see that they approach bipolar disorder by identifying and treating disturbances at the different levels. In keeping with the holism of natural medicine, a number of the therapeutic modalities function on several levels. For example, biological medicine (chapter 4) works on both the Physical and the Electromagnetic Levels, while homeopathy (chapter 9) works on the Mental Level, and Family Systems Therapy (this chapter) works on the Intuitive Level.

The following sections explore the Five Levels of Healing in detail and identify therapies that can remove interference at each level.

The First Level: The Physical Body

The Physical Body includes all the functions on the physical plane, such as the structure and biochemistry of the body. Interference or imbalance at this level can result from an injury or anything that alters the structure, such as accidents, concussions, dental work, or surgery. "Surgery modulates the structure by creating adhesions in the bones and ligaments, which changes the way things act on the Physical Level," says Dr. Klinghardt.

Imbalance at the first level can also result from anything that alters the biochemistry such as poor diet, too much or too little of a nutrient in the diet or in nutritional supplements, or taking the wrong supplements for one's particular biochemistry. Organisms such as bacteria, viruses, and parasites can also change the host's biochemistry. "They all take over the host to some degree and change the host's behavior by modulating its biochemistry," Dr. Klinghardt explains.

"The whole world of toxicity also belongs in the biochemistry," he says. Toxic elements that can alter biochemistry include heavy metals such as mercury, insecticides, pesticides, and other environmental chemicals. Interestingly, heavy metals operate on both the Physical Level and the next level of healing, the Electromagnetic Level. Due to their metallic nature, they can alter the biochemistry by creating electromagnetic disturbances.

In addition, Dr. Klinghardt notes that even if the source of the problem is on the fourth (Intuitive) level, until you get the mercury out, therapies that operate on the fourth level won't be able to clear the interference. The mercury creates a kind of wall that prevents the other therapies from working.

All of these factors at the Physical Level—surgery, injury, dental work, nutritional imbalances, microorganisms, heavy metals and other toxins—can play a role in producing symptoms of mental illness, including bipolar disorder, according to Dr. Klinghardt.

The therapeutic modalities that function at this level are those that address biochemical or structural aspects, from drug and hormone therapies to herbal medicine and nutritional supplements, as well as mechanical therapies such as chiropractic.

The Second Level: The Electromagnetic Body

The Electromagnetic Body is the body's energetic field. Dr. Klinghardt explains it in terms of the traffic of information in the nervous system. "Eighty percent of the messages go up to the brain [from the body], and 20 percent of the messages go down from the brain [to the body]. The nerve currents moving up and down generate a magnetic field that goes out into space, creating an electromagnetic field around the body that interacts with other fields." Acupuncture meridians (energy channels) and the chakra system are part of the Electromagnetic Body.

A chakra, which means 'wheel' in Sanskrit, is an energy vortex or center in the nonphysical counterpart (energy field) of the body. There are seven major chakras positioned roughly from the base of the spine, with points along the spine, to the crown of the head. As with acupuncture meridians, when chakras are blocked, the free flow of energy in the body's field is impeded.

Biophysical stress is a source of disturbance at this level. Biophysical stress is electromagnetic interference from devices that have their own electromagnetic fields, such as electric wall outlets, televisions, microwaves, cell phones, cell phone towers, power lines, and radio stations. These interfere with the electromagnetic system in and around the body.

For example, if you sleep with your head near an electric outlet in the wall, the electromagnetic field from that outlet interferes with your own. An outlet may not even have to be involved. Simply sleeping with your head near a wall in which electric cables run can be sufficient to throw your field off. The brain's blood vessels typically contract in response to the man-made electromagnetic field, leading to decreased blood flow in the brain, says Dr. Klinghardt.

Geopathic stress, or electromagnetic emissions from the Earth, is another source of disturbance. Underground streams and fault lines are a source of these emissions. Again, proximity of your bed to one of these sources—for example, directly over a fault line—can throw your own electromagnetic field out of balance and produce a wide range of symptoms. Simply shifting the position of your bed in the room may remove the problem.

Interference at the second level can cascade down to the Physical Level. The constriction of the blood vessels in the brain in response to biophysical or geopathic stress results in the blood carrying less oxygen and nutrients to the brain. The ensuing deficiencies are a biochemical disturbance, with obvious implications for brain function and mental health. If such deficiencies have their root at the Electromagnetic Level, however, it is important to know that you cannot fix them by taking certain supplements to correct the biochemistry, cautions Dr. Klinghardt.

For example, if an individual has a zinc deficiency, supplementing with zinc may correct the problem if it is merely a biochemical disturbance (a first-level issue). If the restriction of blood flow in the brain as a result of sleeping too close to an electrical outlet (a second-level issue) is behind the deficiency, taking zinc may seem to resolve the problem, but it will return when the person stops taking the supplement. Moving the bed away from the outlet will stop the electromagnetic interference and prevent the recurrence of a zinc deficiency.

Physical trauma or scars can also throw off the second level. "If a scar crosses an acupuncture meridian, it completely alters the energy flow in the system," observes Dr. Klinghardt. An infected tooth or a root canal can accomplish the same. Heavy metal toxicity, from mercury dental fillings and/or environmental metals in the air, water, and food supply, can block the entire electromagnetic system. "We know that the ganglia can be disturbed by a number of things, but toxicity in general is often responsible for throwing off the electromagnetic impulses." Vaccinations can have the same effect. (Ganglia are nerve bundles that are like relay stations for nerve impulses.)

The therapies that address this level of healing are those that correct the distortions of the body's electromagnetic field. Acupuncture and Neural Therapy (see "About the Therapies and Techniques," at the end of the chapter) are two strong modalities for this level. Neural Therapy's injection of local anesthetic in the ganglion breaks up electromagnetic disturbances. You could call the local anesthetic "liquid electricity," says Dr. Klinghardt.

Another therapeutic modality that functions at the second level is Ayurvedic medicine (the traditional medicine of India). As it employs a combination of herbs and energetic interventions, it actually covers the first two levels of healing: the herbs work on the Physical Level, and the energetic aspect on the Electromagnetic Level.

The Third Level: The Mental Body

The third level is the Mental Level or the Mental Body, also known as the Thought Field. This is where your attitudes, beliefs, and early childhood experiences are. "This is the home of psychology," says Dr. Klinghardt. He explains that the Mental Body is outside the Physical Body, rather than housed in the brain. "Memory, thinking, and the mind are all phenomena outside the Physical Body; they are not happening in the brain. The Mental Body is an energetic field."

Disturbances at this level come from traumatic experiences, which can begin as early as conception. Early trauma, or an unresolved conflict situation, leaves faulty circuitry in the Mental Body, explains Dr. Klinghardt. For example, if at two years old, your parents divorced and your father was not allowed by law to see you, you may have formed the beliefs that your father didn't love you and that it was your fault your parents broke up, because you are inherently bad. These damaging beliefs are faulty mental circuitry.

The brain replays traumatic experiences over and over, keeping constant stress signals running through the autonomic nervous system. These disturbances trickle down and affect the Electromagnetic Level of healing, changing nerve function by triggering the constriction of blood vessels, and in turn, affecting the biochemical level in the form of nutritional deficiency.

It may look like a biochemical disturbance, says Dr. Klinghardt, but the cause is much higher up. "Again, this is a situation you cannot treat with lasting results by giving someone supplements, Neural Therapy, or acupuncture." You have to address the third-level interference, the problem in the Mental Body.

Despite what people may conclude from the related names, so-called mental disorders aren't necessarily a function of disturbance in the Mental Body. The cause can be on any of the five levels, iterates Dr. Klinghardt. In fact, in most cases, the third level is not the source. In his experience, most "mental" disorders arise from disturbances on the fourth level. In all cases, the source level must be addressed or a long-term resolution will not be achieved.

Dr. Klinghardt uses Applied Psychoneurobiology, which he developed, to effect healing at the third level (see "About the Therapies and Techniques"). Among the other therapeutic modalities that work at this level are psychotherapy, hypnotherapy, and homeopathy.

The Fourth Level: The Intuitive Body

The fourth level is the Intuitive Body. Some people call it the Dream Body. Experience on this level includes dream states, trance states, and ecstasy, as well as states with a negative association such as nightmares, possession, and curses. The Intuitive Body is what depth psychologist C. G. Jung called the collective unconscious. "On the fourth level, humans are deeply connected with each other and also with flora, fauna, and the global environment," says Dr. Klinghardt.

The fourth level is the realm of shamanism. Other healers who can work at this level to remove interference are those who practice transpersonal psychology. Stated simply, transpersonal refers to an acknowledgment of the phenomena of the fourth level, "the dimension where people are deeply affected by something that isn't of themselves, that is of somebody else. Transpersonal psychology is really a cover-up term for modern shamanism," observes Dr. Klinghardt.

For healing of the Intuitive Body, Dr. Klinghardt uses what is known variously as Family Systems Therapy, Systemic Psychotherapy, or Family Constellation Work. Developed by German psychotherapist Bert Hellinger, the method addresses interference that comes from a previous generation in the family. In this type of interference, says Dr. Klinghardt, "the cause and effect are separated by several generations. It goes over time and space." Rather than a genetic inheritance of a physical weakness, it is an energetic legacy of an injustice with which the family never dealt.

 For more information about Family Systems Therapy and to locate a practitioner, visit the Bert Hellinger website at www.hellinger.com.

The range of specific issues that can be the source is vast, but it usually involves a family member who was excluded in a previous generation. When the other family members don't go through the deep process of grieving the excluded one, whether the exclusion results from separation, death, alienation, or ostracism, the psychic interference of that exclusion is passed on. Another common systemic factor involves identification with victims of a forebear.

"A member of the family two, three, or four generations later will atone for an injustice," without even knowing who the person involved was or what they did, explains Dr. Klinghardt. For example, a woman murders her husband and is never found out. She marries again and lives a long life. Three generations later, one of her great-grandchildren is born. To atone for the murder, the child self-sacrifices by, for example, developing brain cancer at an early age, being abused or murdered, or starting to take drugs as a teenager and committing a slow suicide.

> **Systemic family therapy involves tracing the origins of current illness back to a previous generation. Sometimes an event is known in a family, sometimes it is not. By questioning a client, Dr. Klinghardt is usually able to discover an event from a previous generation that is a likely source of interference for the client's current condition.**

"It's a form of self-punishment that anybody can see on the outside, but nobody understands what is wrong with this child—he had loving parents, good nutrition, went to a good school, and look what he's doing now, he's on drugs. But if you look back two or three generations, you'll see exactly why this child is self-sacrificing." Dr. Klinghardt notes that mental illness is "very often an outcome on the systemic level."

Systemic family therapy involves tracing the origins of current illness back to a previous generation. Sometimes an event is known in a family, sometimes it is not. By questioning a client, Dr. Klinghardt is usually able to discover an event from a previous generation that is a likely source of interference for the client's current condition. If no one knew about a certain event, such as the murder in the example above, there are usually clues in a family that point to those people as a possible source.

For the therapy, the client or a close relative chooses audience members to represent the people in question. In our example, they would be the great-grandmother, great-grandfather, and the new husband. These people come together on a stage or central area. They are not told the story, even when the story is known. "They just go up there not knowing anything, and suddenly feel all these feelings and have all these thoughts come up. . . . Very quickly, within a minute or two, they start feeling like the real people in life have felt, or are feeling in their death now, and start interacting with each other in bizarre ways," says Dr. Klinghardt.

The client typically does not participate, but simply observes. "The therapist does careful therapeutic interventions, but there's very little needed, usually." The person put up for the murdered husband stands there, with no idea of what happened in the past, but then he falls to the floor. When someone asks, "What happened to you?" he answers, "I've been murdered." It just comes out of his mouth. Then the therapist asks if he wants to say anything to any of the other people. He speaks to his wife and it becomes clear that she was the one who murdered him. They speak back and forth, and "very quickly, there's deep healing that happens between the two," states Dr. Klinghardt. "Usually we relive the pain and the truth that was there . . . It's very, very dramatic . . . Then the therapist does some healing therapeutic intervention with those representatives."

Family Systems Therapy is not a long-term endeavor. Dr. Klinghardt has found that the releasing work can be completed

> ## In Their Own Words
>
> "You can't just hand a bipolar person lithium and be done with her. I mean, you can—and that's exactly what is done for most bipolar people. But that's not treatment. That's not good care."[169]
>
> —Lizzie Simon, bipolar at 17, author of *Detour*

rapidly, usually in one to three sessions. "The remarkable thing about the systemic work is that it is so quick," he says.

With removal of the interference that was transmitted down the generations, the client's condition is resolved, although the trickle-down effect to the lower levels of healing may need to be addressed. Often, however, healing at the higher level is sufficient. With balance restored at that level, the other levels are then able to correct themselves.

Dr. Klinghardt likens Family Systems Therapy to shamanic work in Africa, in which healing often has to be done from a distance through a representative because of the impracticability of having a sick child, for example, traveling 200 miles from the village to see the medicine man. The representative holds a piece of clothing or hair from that child, and the shaman does the healing work on the stranger. "There's a magical effect broadcast back to the child," says Dr. Klinghardt. "The child often gets well. It's the same principle [with Family Systems Therapy]. We call it surrogate healing." He adds that Systemic Family Therapy has become very popular in Europe in the last two years, while it is still relatively new in the United States.

Dr. Klinghardt has developed a variation of this technique that enables the work to happen with just a practitioner and the patient in a regular treatment room. He accomplishes the same end without representatives of the antecedents, using Autonomic Response Testing (ART, a kind of muscle testing; see "About the Therapies and Techniques") to pinpoint what happened and engage in the dialogues that arise in this work.

He gives the example of a 45-year-old woman who had lived daily with asthma from the time she was two years old. Through ART, in a kind of process of elimination, Dr. Klinghardt learned that physical causes were not the source of the asthma and that it had to do with exclusion of some kind in a previous generation. Further exploration revealed that this woman's mother had lost a younger sibling when she was two years old. In this case, the woman knew of the event, but that was all she knew. ART confirmed the connection between this buried information and the asthma. Dr. Klinghardt stopped the session at this point, instructing his client to find out what she could about this family occurrence and then come back.

The woman's mother was still alive and told her that the baby died shortly after birth, was buried behind the house without a gravestone or other marker on the site, and was never mentioned again in the family. Everyone knew where the child was buried, but there was an unspoken agreement never to speak of her. Not only that, but the next child born was given the same name, as if the one who had died had never existed or, worse, had been replaced.

"This was a violation of a principle of what we know about Systemic Family Therapy, which is that each member that's born into a family has the same and equal right to belong to the family," said Dr. Klinghardt. Exclusion, even in memory, is a form of injustice, and creates interference energy that is transmitted through the generations. Exclusion of a family member in the past is frequently the source of disturbance at the Intuitive Level, according to Dr. Klinghardt.

The client came back for the second session, and Dr. Klinghardt put her into a light trance state. "In that trance state she was able to contact that being, the dead sibling, and say to her, 'I remember you now, I bring you back into my family, I give you a place in my heart, I will never forget you,' he relates. Then she cried, and it was a very transformative experience." He observes that this process required very little guidance from him and took only about 20 minutes.

During the session, the woman made a commitment to go back to the house where the child was buried—it was still a family property—and put a gravestone on her grave. After the session, the woman's asthma was clearly better. She rated it at 50 to 60 percent better, and reported later that it stayed that way. "It took her about three months to put up the gravestone, and she said the day after she set up the gravestone for that child, her asthma disappeared completely," relates Dr. Klinghardt. That was eight years ago, and the asthma has not returned.

Dr. Klinghardt and others who practice Family Systems Therapy have seen similar connections in cases of mental illness.

Bipolar disorder, chronic anxiety or depression, schizophrenia, addiction, hyperactivity in children, aggressive behavior, and autism can all lead back to systemic family issues. In fact, Dr. Klinghardt estimates that "about 70 percent of mental disorders across the board go back to systemic family issues that need to be treated. People try to treat them psychologically, on the third level, and it cannot work. This is not the right level." Similarly, focusing on the biochemistry is not going to fix the problem when the source is at the fourth level.

The Fifth Level: The Spiritual

The fifth level is the direct relationship of the patient with God, or whatever name you choose for the divine. Interference in this relationship can be caused by early childhood experiences, past-life traumas, or enlightenment experiences with a guru or other spiritual teacher. Of the latter, Dr. Klinghardt says, "Some enlightenment experiences actually turn out to be a block. If the experience occurred in context with a guru, the person may become unable to reach there without the guru. The very thing that showed them what to look for becomes an obstacle."

This level requires self-healing when there is separation or interference in a person's connection to the divine. Direct contact with nature is one way to reforge the connection. "True prayer and true meditation work on this level as ways of getting there, but it's a level where there is no possibility of interaction between the healer and the patient," states Dr. Klinghardt. "I always say, if anybody tries to be helpful on this level, run as fast as you can." He notes that gurus and other spiritual teachers belong on the fourth level and have a valuable place there, but have no business on the fifth level. If they trespass into that level, they are putting themselves where God should be, says Dr. Klinghardt. "It's very dangerous."

That said, a number of the therapies in this book clear impediments to spiritual connection at other levels, thus opening the way for individuals to reestablish balance for themselves on the fifth level.

Natural Medicine and the Five Levels of Healing

The chart below shows on what level the natural medicine therapeutic modalities in this book function.

Therapy	Level	Chapter
Anthroposophic Medicine	Mental Body Spiritual Body	4
Applied Psychoneurobiology	Physical Body Electromagnetic Body Mental Body	3
Biological Medicine	Physical Body Electromagnetic Body	4
Cranial Osteopathy	Physical Body Electromagnetic Body	7
Family Systems Therapy	Intuitive Body	3, 7
Homeopathy	Mental Body	9
NAET (allergy elimination)	Electromagnetic Body	8
Neural Therapy	Electromagnetic Body	3
Nutritional/Dietary Therapy	Physical Body	3–6
Shamanic Healing	Intuitive Body	10

Operating Principles of the Five Healing Levels

The levels affect each other differently, depending on whether the influence is traveling upward or downward. Both trauma and successful therapeutic intervention at the higher levels have a rapid and deeply penetrating effect on the lower levels, says Dr. Klinghardt. This means that both the cause and the cure at the upper levels spread downward quickly. For example, if a systemic family issue is strongly present at the fourth (Intuitive) level, it will have profound effects on the first three levels. Similarly, resolving that issue can produce rapid changes in the Physical, Electromagnetic, and Mental Bodies. The lower levels may correct on their own, without further remediation.

At the same time, trauma or therapeutic intervention at the lower levels has a very slow, and little penetrating, effect upwards. When you get a physical injury (the first level), for instance, it will gradually change your electromagnetic field (the second level), altering the energy flow in your body. It's a slow process, however. The same is true for healing. "If you want to heal an injury on the second level, let's say you have a chakra that's blocked, you can do that by giving herbs and vitamins—biochemical interventions—but it will take years," says Dr. Klinghardt. But if you do an intervention on the third or fourth level, it can correct the blocked chakra on the second level immediately, within seconds or minutes, he notes.

Bipolar Disorder and the Five Levels of Healing

As stated earlier, bipolar disorder can be the result of interference or disturbance on any of the Five Levels of Healing. In his practice, Dr. Klinghardt has discovered certain trends, however. "Bipolar is, for me, interesting in that it has very few elements on the second (Electromagnetic) level, is fairly strong on the third (Mental) level, but really strong on the fourth (Intuitive) and on the first (Physical)," he says.

Bipolar and the Physical Level

The Physical Level elements most often involved in bipolar disorder are nutritional factors, an imbalance of intestinal flora, and viruses, says Dr. Klinghardt. As discussed in chapter 2, certain nutritional deficiencies, notably of essential fatty acids, seem to be associated with bipolar disorder—witness the effectiveness of fish oil and other EFA supplementation in reducing or eliminating symptoms. In Dr. Klinghardt's experience, the stabilizing effect of these supplements alone can be quite dramatic.

As poor diet and digestion can be the source of nutritional deficiencies, it is essential to address these factors in treatment. No one diet works for everyone because people process foods differently. To determine the optimum diet for an individual, Dr.

Klinghardt uses metabolic typing, a scientific method that identifies a person's particular metabolism and prescribes a diet that works best for the way that person processes food.

 For more information on metabolic typing, see *The Metabolic Typing Diet,* by William L. Wolcott (Doubleday, 2000).

Compromised digestion has significance beyond potential nutritional deficiencies. Bipolar disorder shares with autism a strong connection between intestinal health and brain function, observes Dr. Klinghardt (see "Intestinal Dysbiosis" in chapter 2 of this book and the author's *The Natural Medicine Guide to Autism*). In both cases, the microorganisms in the bowel are out of balance and contribute to the symptoms that characterize the disorders. In bipolar disorder, the imbalance is implicated in frequent manic episodes. The microorganism involved is typically the bacterium *Clostridium,* which is normally present in the intestines but due to a variety of factors (such as a chronically poor diet and repeated use of antibiotics) multiplies beyond its normal levels.

To restore intestinal balance, the main remedy Dr. Klinghardt employs is garlic. He calls it a "magic tool" for this purpose. "Garlic contains a large number of highly antibacterial, antifungal, and antiviral compounds, and it completely changes the bowel flora over time," says Dr. Klinghardt. "We also use garlic to increase the microcirculation in the brain, as it works as a blood thinner." To gain these beneficial effects, garlic must be taken after a meal, not on an empty stomach. With his patients, he uses freeze-dried garlic, which is inexpensive and has much less odor. The dosage is two capsules (750 mg each) three times daily, after each meal. "I do not recommend raw garlic, since the quality and amount of active ingredients depend on the soil in which it is grown."

The noncompliance problem that is so frequently cited in psychiatric circles regarding patients and medications for bipolar disorder does not seem to be an issue with this protocol. "We have people doing so much better within two months of this, that they miss the garlic if they don't take it," he reports.

In addition to the garlic and dietary measures that improve digestion, Dr. Klinghardt supplements with probiotics, beneficial intestinal bacteria such as acidophilus that also help restore the balance of flora. He notes that probiotics must be taken after a meal, not before it, or they will not survive to help repopulate the gut.

The good news is that changing the bowel flora is "fairly easy," according to Dr. Klinghardt. "You get the nutrition right, you feed them garlic, you feed them healthy bowel flora, and, without any use of antibiotics, the bowel flora will normalize. Within two months, people start having signs of improvement."

The other factor on the Physical Level that is often present in bipolar disorder, and schizophrenia as well, is an underlying virus, says Dr. Klinghardt. The presence of a virus is determined through Autonomic Response Testing (see "About the Therapies and Techniques"). The viruses are often contracted in the womb, transmitted from the mother to the fetus, and tend to be herpes viruses, such as genital herpes or herpes simplex (the virus that causes cold sores).

The mere presence of the virus in the body is not problematic in itself. It is when the virus is able to replicate that problems begin. In order to replicate, viral particles must be able to penetrate into new cells. Healthy cell membranes in the body prevent this from occurring. As cell membranes are made up of oils, such as essential fatty acids, the EFA deficiency characteristic of bipolar disorder has serious consequences. The compromised cell membranes in people with an EFA deficiency allow the viral load to rise.

This may still not be a problem until other factors combine to create an overload on the body's nervous and other systems that then manifests as bipolar disorder or schizophrenia. The rapid hormonal changes of the teen years may be one of the factors that in combination with the virus serve to trigger these disorders. This is a possible explanation for why these two mental illnesses typically have their onset in early adulthood.

Fortunately, it is a relatively simple matter to stabilize the system, says Dr. Klinghardt. EFA supplementation—he uses mainly fish and coconut oils—is actually a powerful antiviral measure in that it strengthens the cell membranes and in so doing suppresses viral replication in the body. *Uña de gato* (cat's claw), a South American herb, is another strong antiviral, as is the herb cilantro. The latter is also a natural chelator, meaning it gets heavy metals such as mercury out of the body, which has additional benefit for people with bipolar disorder (see "About the Therapies and Techniques").

Heavy metal detoxification in itself has not shown as strong therapeutic results with bipolar disorder as it has with other disorders, such as depression, for example, but "it is important with all psychiatric and neurological illnesses that people have a metal-free mouth," says Dr. Klinghardt, referring to mercury fillings and other metal-containing dental items. The leaching of mercury from fillings is an ongoing source of exposure to a known neurotoxin. "In terms of mental illness, probably the more important effect is that each metal has a strong electromagnetic field around it. The upper teeth are close to the brain. The field of metal crowns, metal fillings, and metal bridges impairs the blood flow inside the brain, and that's a very important thing with all the mental illnesses."

The fact that lithium, which is a metal, is used to treat bipolar disorder suggests to Dr. Klinghardt that "a disturbance in the metal metabolism of the body underlies it." This makes it all the more important to remove the sources of heavy metal toxicity from the body to reduce the body's exposure. Without correcting the metabolic problem, however, detoxification methods such as chelation are unlikely to be of lasting benefit, as a body compromised in this way is unable to eliminate the heavy metals to which the body will inevitably be reexposed in our toxic environment.

 For more about dysfunction in metal metabolism, see chapter 5.

A word of caution is necessary at this point. Mercury filling removal needs to be done by a dentist who has been trained in how to do this safely and effectively, as mercury vapors and particles are released during the removal process.

Resources For information about dental mercury, see the websites of Dr. Joseph Mercola at www.mercola.com and Dental Amalgam Mercury Syndrome (DAMS) at www.dams.cc. For help in locating a dentist, call the DAMS National Office at 800-311-6265.

Bipolar Disorder and the Electromagnetic Level

In most cases, Dr. Klinghardt finds that there is not much involvement of the Electromagnetic Level in bipolar disorder. "We look at the sleeping location in relation to the wires in the wall," he says. "But it isn't as predominant a factor as it is in other mental disorders." Nevertheless, it is a good idea for everyone to consider the proximity of their bed to an electric outlet or whether it is positioned over a fault line or underground stream and resituate the bed to avoid these influences.

Again, biophysical or geopathic stress amplifies the symptoms of heavy metal toxicity, says Dr. Klinghardt. Heavy metals are found mostly in the brain, where they work like antennae, he explains. They pick up the electromagnetic or geopathic interference, which exacerbates the symptoms of mental disorders. Repositioning the bed can eliminate this exacerbating effect.

While disturbances at the Electromagnetic Level tend not to be a major factor in bipolar disorder, Dr. Klinghardt did have one patient for whom such disturbances were actually the source of his condition. As noted previously, scars can throw off the energy flow in the body. In the case of this man, Dr. Klinghardt discovered that the scars of a childhood tonsillectomy were creating an energy interference. Neural therapy injections in the scarred region corrected the problem and the bipolar symptoms and episodes disappeared and did not return after that. Aside from that case, Dr. Klinghardt reports that he hasn't observed much success with acupuncture and neural therapy as bipolar disorder treatment.

Bipolar Disorder and the Mental Level

In considering the contribution of third-level (Mental Body) factors, Dr. Klinghardt looks for early childhood trauma.

Generally, the trauma occurs later than it does in cases of depression, which can involve trauma as far back as conception, he says. In bipolar disorder, the trauma usually occurs between the ages of two and six years and involves a separation of some sort such as the death of a parent or divorce.

"On the Mental Level in cases of bipolar disorder, we often find a lot of unresolved childhood material, often in a similar setup to that of schizophrenia," says Dr. Klinghardt. This setup is that the child is torn in alliance between warring parents— "Should I align myself with my dad, or should I align myself with my mom?" Psychotherapy can help get at these issues, and insight may bring some improvement, but generally not complete recovery.

Bipolar Disorder and the Intuitive Level

On the fourth (Intuitive) level, however, profound healing is possible. In Dr. Klinghardt's experience, intervention on this and the first level produces the greatest results with bipolar disorder because these are the two levels most often implicated and with the greatest degree of disturbance.

Again, he has found that the pattern in bipolar disorder in the arena of family systems is similar to schizophrenia. The typical pattern in both is that the child identifies with more than one person from a previous generation. Or stated in another way, "the child is strongly identified with two completely different consciousness fields," explains Dr. Klinghardt. "One person was abused in a certain way, and another one was excluded or abused in another way. There aren't enough offspring to take this on, and it all ends up in one person. That person develops two different streams of consciousness."

He gives the example of a grandfather who fought in Vietnam and participated in killing the children in a village. He also became involved with a Vietnamese woman, got her pregnant, and then abandoned her. Later, the man married and had only one child who also had only one child, a son.

"Now, two generations later, there's one offspring, but two generations before there are two victims: the village children and the woman who was left with another child. The one offspring, the grandchild, has the job of atoning for both the massacre in the village and for the illegitimate child that wasn't recognized, that wasn't nurtured. The grandchild will unconsciously be identified with the victims in the village, and behave like a child who has been murdered or crippled by machine-gun fire or Agent Orange or whatever it was. The child at the same time will behave as if it is an abandoned child whose father has disappeared. That split of being identified with two different consciousness fields at the same time in the same person, we very often find, is the cause of schizophrenia or bipolar disorder."

Through Family Systems Therapy, the dually identified person can make peace with the ancestors or victims and release the need to atone. As mentioned previously, this is not a long-term therapy, but can be accomplished in one to three sessions. The following case illustrates the process.

Frederick: Ten Years of Bipolar Disorder

Frederick, 35, had suffered from bipolar disorder and been taking lithium off and on since he was 25. A scientist who designed electrical equipment, he was regarded as brilliant in his field. "When he was in his manic phase, he invented incredible things and was a genius on the piano," recalls Dr. Klinghardt. "But he would also hire a taxi to drive 600 miles or buy a new piano when he had no credit left." With characteristic charm, he was able to convince the seller that he would come back the next day and pay for the piano, and the seller would allow him to take the instrument home. Displaying the lavish spending habits that often accompany mania, he made numerous such large purchases and amassed huge debt. His manic phase typically lasted over a month and cost him around $100,000.

When he plunged into depression, as he invariably did, his doctor would put him back on lithium. On the drug, Frederick gained weight and couldn't work. He felt devoid of ideas and was not productive; at these times, he was in danger of losing his job. Eventually, unable to endure that state any longer, he would go off the lithium again, and return to creativity at work and spending too much. Since he went through two or three cycles of mania and depression per year, the consequences to his life were severe. He came to Dr. Klinghardt looking for a way to stop the vicious circle.

ART revealed a viral load and high mercury levels. Dr. Klinghardt immediately started Frederick on the freeze-dried garlic at the dosage cited earlier and EPA (eicosapentaenoic acid), an omega-3 essential fatty acid derived from fish oil, at a dosage of 360 mg in capsule form four times a day. Dr. Klinghardt notes that, although 2000 mg a day is optimal, the dosage of around 1500 mg that Frederick took is about the most people can tolerate due to the unpleasant taste from burping up fish oil. As oral mercury chelation, Frederick took twenty drops of cilantro per day.

At the same time, Dr. Klinghardt implemented a method called enhancement technique, which consists of acupressure to the tip of the middle finger on both hands. (Acupressure works like acupuncture, except light manual pressure is used in place of needles to stimulate acupoints, which are the points on the channels or meridians along which energy travels throughout the body.) The right middle finger corresponds to the right side of the brain and the left middle finger to the left side of the brain. Stimulating the acupoint on each increases the blood flow to the brain, he explains. "This allows the substances that you give orally to accumulate selectively in the brain, to concentrate there." Dr. Klinghardt showed Frederick how to do the enhancement technique, so he could perform it himself four times daily on both hands.

As dietary measures, Dr. Klinghardt recommended a high-protein, low-carbohydrate diet and the elimination of all grains, sugar and other sweets, and aspartame. (Metabolic typing was not yet available.)

On this program, Frederick was able to undergo a careful withdrawal from lithium over the next year. Dr. Klinghardt very slowly tapered it down and finally stopped it completely. Frederick had no manic recurrence during that time. He stayed mildly depressed, however, even when he was completely off the lithium, which was significant because for the previous ten years whenever he went off the drug, he would become manic.

Fourteen months after starting treatment with Dr. Klinghardt, Frederick had still not had a manic episode, but he remained depressed. At that point, Dr. Klinghardt turned to Family Systems Therapy. Through ART and Applied Psychoneurobiology, they learned that Frederick had the characteristic dual identification of many people with bipolar disorder.

On one side, there was his maternal grandfather, who had been a Nazi involved in the murder of Jews. Frederick was identified with the victims. In fact, when he was not on lithium, he looked like a Holocaust victim, recalls Dr. Klinghardt. "He was skinny, pale, fragile-looking, and bent over like the photographs of the Jews in European ghettos. He even dressed like that, always in black. So on one side he was identified with being a murdered Jew or someone in the ghetto at least, though he wasn't Jewish."

On the other side was Frederick's father, who early in Frederick's life was ousted by his wife and family when they discovered that he was bisexual. None of them ever heard from him again. So on this side Frederick was identified with his father who was pushed out of the family.

Frederick was an only child and, in fact, the only offspring on both sides of the family. As a result, the need for atonement on both sides of the family was concentrated in this one person.

Family Systems Therapy is based on the premise "that each member has an equal right to belong," says Dr. Klinghardt. That means that bisexuality is not grounds for exclusion. "It's all right for the wife to divorce her husband because of his sexual orientation, but it's not all right for her to forbid him all contact with their child."

In identifying with two different people, in this instance the maternal grandfather and the father, "one side of the brain is behaving like this person, and the other side of the brain is behaving like that person. You get confused. It's a setup for bipolar development." In some people, the mania and depression metaphorically reflect what happened in previous generations, Dr. Klinghardt observes.

In Frederick's case, he was identified with his father at both poles of his disorder. When depressed, he withdrew from life and pushed people away, including his family. In the manic state, he might be charming and gregarious, but the mania was a barrier between him and others, and served to push people away as much as his depression did. It was as if Frederick was doing to himself what was done to his father.

After learning what had happened in the family, Dr. Klinghardt gave Frederick the homework assignment of reading books about the Holocaust, including firsthand accounts by survivors, so he would understand what happened and get a clear picture of what it was like for Jews and others targeted for extermination. With that knowledge, he was ready to atone for the actions of his grandfather and release the need for identification with the victims.

As often happens in Family Systems Therapy, it took only one session for Frederick to release his dual identification. "We had him bow to the killed Jews, acknowledge them deeply in a heartfelt way." To let go of his identification with his father, he needed to acknowledge his father and restore him to his rightful place in the family. He spoke to him in the session, saying, "Dad, you know you're my father, you're the right father for me. Even though you were bisexual, you're still my father and I give you a place in my life."

Frederick tried to find his father, but was unsuccessful. His family had always focused on the story of how his father was "perverted." He pressed them for other details and learned that his father was a talented artist who had created a beautiful home for the family and done a lot of good things. Between the Family Systems work and seeing that his father was not the bad person he had been portrayed to be, Frederick was able to form a bond with his father within himself.

After the Family Systems session, Frederick's depression lifted. At that point, Dr. Klinghardt advised him to reduce his EPA dosage to a maintenance schedule of 180 mg three times a day. He also had him start on evening primrose oil, an omega-6 essential fatty acid, to balance the omega-3 fish oil and his chemistry. Three years after he came to Dr. Klinghardt for treatment, Frederick had still had no recurrence of manic or depressive episodes.

About the Therapies and Techniques

Applied Psychoneurobiology (APN): This therapeutic technique was developed by Dr. Klinghardt. Employing his muscle testing method (see "Autonomic Response Testing," which follows) as a guide, APN uses stress signals in the autonomic nervous system to communicate with a patient's unconscious mind. "You can establish a code with the unconscious mind for yes and no in answer to questions," he explains. "The code is the strength or the weakness of a test muscle." APN can lead the way to the beliefs that underlie illness such as bipolar disorder, and exchange those beliefs with ones that promote balance in the Mental Body. This can produce dramatic shifts in the health and well-being of the person, notes Dr. Klinghardt.

Autonomic Response Testing (ART): ART, also called neural kinesiology, is a system of testing developed by Dr. Klinghardt. It employs a variety of methods, including muscle response testing and arm length testing, to measure changes in the autonomic nervous system. (The autonomic nervous system controls the automatic processes of the body such as respiration, heart rate, digestion, and response to stress.) ART is used to identify distress in the body and determine optimum treatment.

In general, a strong arm (or finger, depending on the kind of muscle testing) or an even arm length (in arm length testing) indicates that the system is not in distress. A weak muscle or uneven arm length indicates the presence of a factor that is causing stress to the client's organism.

Chelation: This is a therapy that removes heavy metals from the body, among other therapeutic functions. DMPS (2,3-dimercaptopropane-1-sulfonate) is a substance used as a chelating agent, which means that it binds with heavy metals, notably mercury, and is then excreted from the body. DMPS can be administered orally, intravenously, or intramuscularly. Other chelation agents are cilantro, chlorella, alpha lipoic acid, and glutathione.

Neural therapy: Developed by German physicians in 1925, neural therapy employs the injection of local anesthetics such as procaine into specific sites in the body to clear interferences in the flow of electrical energy and restore proper nerve function. The interferences, or "interference fields" as they are known in the profession, can be the result of a scar, other old injury, physical trauma, or dental conditions such as root-canalled or impacted teeth, all of which have their own energy fields that can disrupt the body's normal energy flow.

Disruption in the body's energy field has far-flung effects, and can manifest in seemingly unrelated conditions. "Any part of the body that has been traumatized or ill—no matter where it is located—can become an interference field which may cause disturbance anywhere in the body," states Dr. Klinghardt.[170] Neural therapy injections may be into glands, acupuncture points, or ganglia (nerve bundles that are like relay stations for nerve impulses), as well as scars or sites of trauma.

For more information about the therapies or to locate a practitioner near you, see the following:

APN, ART, and Neural therapy: Dr. Klinghardt (see appendix B); websites: www.neuraltherapy.com and www.pnf.org/neural_kinesiology.html.

Chelation: The American College for Advancement in Medicine (ACAM), 23121 Verdugo Drive, Suite 204, Laguna Hills, CA 92653; fax: 949-455-9679; website: www.acam.org.

4 Healing from a Cellular to a Spiritual Level: Biological Medicine

"In my opinion, everybody coming to see me is a psychiatric patient," says Bradford S. Weeks, M.D., whose practice is based in Clinton, Washington. "By this I mean that everyone has compounding spiritual issues that affect the soul and the physical body. I don't make a distinction between psychiatric illnesses and other illnesses."

Dr. Weeks' medical training is both extensive and an unusual combination. He specializes in the sophisticated discipline of biological medicine, with a focus on anthroposophic medicine. His conventional medical study was in two particularly rigorous fields, neurology and psychiatry. Now his practice (and the workshops, seminars, and lectures he regularly delivers around the country) is devoted to addressing the body, mind, and spirit components of illness—in other words, to treating his patients holistically.

What Is Biological Medicine?

Biological medicine is based on the principle that illness is a reflection of imbalance in the body, and imbalance in one part affects the whole. Multiple factors, such as diet, psychological stress, toxic exposure (to heavy metals, chemicals, or radiation, or the overuse of pharmaceuticals), intestinal disturbances, and immune system overload, can disturb the natural balance in the body. Thus far, biological medicine is similar to other holistic medical approaches.

What distinguishes biological medicine from these other approaches is that biological medicine identifies disturbances in the natural balance of the body down to the tissue and cellular level, where dysfunctional patterns can be seen (often before they manifest in symptoms). In other words, the multiple factors cited can throw your cellular function out of whack, which in turn generates the symptoms of illness if balance is not restored.

The disturbances in cellular, tissue, and organ function can be identified and remedied. Since cellular function is at the root of all action in the body, restoring balance at the cellular and connective tissue level restores the balance of all body systems and helps the body improve its regulatory functions and its natural ability to heal itself. Thus, looking at the biological (cellular and tissue) terrain of the body, the "internal milieu" as it is known in biological medicine, goes to the roots of illness. Biological medicine relies on special blood, urine, and saliva tests to assess the internal milieu.

To restore the chemistry and internal balance of the body, biological medicine draws from a wide range of therapeutic modalities. A biological medicine physician may employ dietary changes, nutritional supplements, enzyme therapy, detoxification techniques, phytotherapy (herbal medicine), anthroposophic medicine, acupuncture/traditional Chinese medicine, neural therapy, CranioSacral therapy, heat treatments, and/or homeopathy. The latter may consist of classical homeopathy; combination formulas; drainage remedies that improve organ and tissue capacity to drain toxicities from the body; or preparations called Sanum remedies, which are formulas developed by Dr. Guenther Enderlein, a German bacteriologist and microbiologist whose work in the early decades of the twentieth century became a cornerstone of biological medicine.

Detoxification is another important component of biological medicine treatment. If the body is overloaded with toxins, cellular integrity is compromised, and the dysfunction of organs and systems will follow if the load is not reduced. Many diseases, including cancer, are diseases of toxicity.

Biological dentistry is also a vital facet of biological medicine. Dental factors, such as mercury toxicity from fillings, root canals, and chronic asymptomatic jawbone infections, are primary causes of disturbance in the body. Biological dentistry recognizes that problems in the teeth can create problems throughout the body, both through blockage of energy and the spread of infection. Correcting teeth and jaw problems is therefore essential in restoring health.

As a holistic medicine, biological medicine regards psychological and spiritual factors as important as physical factors in the creation of illness and the restoration of health. Thus, psychological and spiritual counseling are often part of biological medicine treatment, as is anthroposophic medicine.

Anthroposophic medicine, developed in the 1920s by Austrian scientist Rudolf Steiner, is based upon the view that humans are spiritual beings and the body cannot be treated separately from the spirit. The medicines, which are an extension of homeopathic remedies, address the spiritual aspect of a patient. Anthroposophic medicine is widely practiced in Europe, and the number of practitioners in the United States is increasing.

Biological medicine originated in Europe, arising from Dr. Enderlein's theory of pleomorphism, which is in direct opposition to the germ theory advanced by Louis Pasteur in the late 1800s and embraced by conventional Western medicine. In contrast to the view held by the germ theory that bacteria and other microorganisms invade us from without to cause illness, pleomorphism holds that these microbes already exist in us. It is when they change shape (morph), moving through many (pleo) shapes, due to biochemical alterations in the internal milieu of the body, that they produce disease.

Good health depends upon our coexisting in harmony with the millions of microorganisms in our bodies (a state called symbiosis). The toxicities and stress of modern life, and attendant deficiencies, disturb this balance (dysbiosis) and lead to illness if the imbalance is allowed to continue. With pleomorphism as its base, the emphasis in biological medicine is on monitoring the cellular terrain and maintaining or restoring its balance to both prevent and reverse illness.

Some practitioners in the United States are now using the term biological medicine to describe a range of holistic therapies, which may not reflect the mission and focus of the biological medicine that originated in Europe. Those who are rooted in the European tradition of biological medicine, with its focus on cellular terrain, the internal milieu, and the other principles just delineated, use the term "European biological medicine" to designate that alliance and practice.

Biological medicine begins by identifying what is happening in the body on a cellular level. Treatment is not a matter of simply substituting an herb or other natural medicine for a prescription medication. Regardless of the natural medicine used, this is "still thinking like conventional medicine," says Thomas Rau, M.D., a pioneer in European biological medicine. A comprehensive and accurate approach to treatment, which reflects the quite different orientation of biological medicine to health and healing, is to determine exactly what is occurring in the cellular terrain, and then to begin there "to clean and to build up the milieu."

For information about and referral to practitioners of biological medicine, contact the Biological Medicine Network, c/o Marion Foundation, 3 Barnabas Road, Marion, MA 02738: 508-748-0816; E-mail: bmn@marionfoundation.org. For information about anthroposophic medicine, see the Anthroposophic Press; P.O. Box 960, Herndon, VA 20172-0960; tel: 703-661-1594 or 800-856-8664; website: www.anthropress.org. For referral to practitioners, contact the Physicians' Association for Anthroposophical Medicine (PAAM), 1923 Geddes Avenue, Ann Arbor, MI 48104-1797; tel: 734-930-9462; website: www.paam.net.

From Cell to Spirit

From Dr. Weeks' perspective, bipolar disorder involves imbalance in what is known in anthroposophic medicine and other traditions as the four harmonious members of the human body: the physical body, the etheric body, the astral body, and the spirit. (These correspond to the Physical, Electromagnetic, Intuitive, and Spiritual levels, respectively, in Dr. Klinghardt's model of healing described in the previous chapter.) This imbalance can be seen as a dis-ease or disharmony between the four. In Dr. Weeks' experience, correcting imbalances at the physical level alone can produce excellent results with bipolar disorder. However, he encourages his patients to consider the psychological and spiritual components of their condition as well.

The Physical Level

In treatment, Dr. Weeks starts with the physical because there are typically biochemical imbalances that can stop the mood swings relatively quickly when corrected. The first step is to run blood tests such as a red blood cell essential fatty acid profile and amino acid profile to identify specific deficiencies and design a treatment plan accordingly. Initially, it is also important to eliminate an under- or overactive thyroid as a factor, as both can produce bipolar manifestations, notes Dr. Weeks.

At this stage, it's also a good idea to consider whether allergies or, more accurately, food sensitivities or intolerances are playing a role. "Most of what are called food allergies are really food intolerances," he says. "If you enhance the digestive enzymes or reduce the amount of wheat and dairy and so forth, then the person does well with digesting it." In Dr. Weeks' experience, "most mentally ill patients are dairy intolerant." As discussed in chapter 2, food intolerances can affect the brain and behavior, thus the term "brain allergies."

 For more about allergies and how to identify and eliminate them, see chapter 8.

While everyone is different and treatment needs to be individualized according to test results and other factors, there are certain conditions that are frequently present in bipolar disorder at the physical level, according to Dr. Weeks. They are hypoglycemia, dehydration, GABA dysfunction, essential fatty acid deficiency, and amino acid deficiency.

Hypoglycemia: "It is critically important to control hypoglycemia in bipolar patients. Most are hypoglycemic," says Dr. Weeks. "People just have coffee and doughnuts for breakfast, then they crash, and they have another coffee and doughnut. That can really exacerbate bipolar disorder." Eating nutritionally balanced meals and avoiding coffee and fast-burning carbohydrates can help prevent hypoglycemia.

Water: "The number one issue for people with bipolar disorder is dehydration," Dr. Weeks states. "Almost without exception they're dehydrated. They're doing Pepsi, Coke, sugar, coffee. These are all things that lead to net water loss. Water is a buffer and a solvent. When people are adequately hydrated, things are calmer. When they're not adequately hydrated, people run more acidically. Electrolytes are a little imbalanced. Nothing quite fires correctly."

Dr. Weeks tells his patients to drink half their weight in ounces of bottled or filtered water daily. This means that if you weigh 150 pounds, you should drink 75 ounces of water a day. It is best not to drink the water with meals as it dilutes digestive stomach acids and enzymes, he says. He advises keeping bottles of water by the bed and in the bathroom, so you can drink 16 ounces of water as soon as you wake up in the morning and another 16 ounces when you brush your teeth. He tells his patients to treat it "like it's heart medication. Just as most of us get heart attacks first thing in the morning and it's hardest to start your car in the morning, our most stressful time biochemically is first thing in the morning. That's when you really need to be well hydrated."

GABA: GABA (gamma-aminobutyric acid) is an amino acid that also acts as a neurotransmitter. It exerts a calming effect on the brain. People with bipolar disorder typically have a deficiency of GABA and a dysfunction of some kind in their GABA receptor sites, says Dr. Weeks. Certain substances, including alcohol and the tranquilizers Valium and Klonopin, stimulate GABA receptors, he explains, adding that "back rubs and massage, nice music and lullabies" do so as well. GABA can be taken as an amino acid supplement to promote GABA's calming influence on the brain. However, "if the receptors don't work, plenty of GABA won't help," Dr. Weeks notes.

Essential Fatty Acids: Dr. Weeks assumes unless it is proven otherwise that his patients with bipolar disorder are deficient in essential fatty acids, specifically the omega-3s. A simple blood test, called the red blood cell membrane essential fatty acid panel, confirms this. "It's also easy to test by asking about the person's dietary history," he notes. If McDonald's French fries and other junk foods containing trans-fatty acids feature prominently in the diet, then EFA deficiency is more than likely, he explains. As discussed in chapter 2, trans-fatty acids interfere with EFA metabolism in the body.

To illustrate the role of EFAs in mood regulation, Dr. Weeks turns to an ancient sailing practice. "In the old days, when sailors were coming into a seaport, they would slash open a keg of whale oil and throw some on the water because the wind can get no purchase on the waves that way. While the wind can still blow, the oil slick in the harbor made the waves drop so they could cruise into a safe anchorage. Oil has the same effect on the brain."

Fish oil supplementation demonstrates this effect on mood. "Oils can be considered a first-line, stand-alone therapy for bipolar disorder," states Dr. Weeks.

Amino Acids: Deficiency in amino acid precursors to neurotransmitters is another common feature in bipolar disorder. Amino acid supplementation is typically part of the protocol for bipolar disorder. Tryptophan, its close relative 5-HTP, and tyrosine supplements provide the precursors for the "feel good" neurotransmitters.

As amino acids are the building blocks of protein, people are usually deficient in B vitamins as well. Dr. Weeks has found intramuscular injections of vitamins in the B complex family, with a special emphasis on vitamin B_{12} and folic acid, to be "very, very helpful in calming people down." He teaches his patients how to administer the shots themselves so they are not dependent on him and can reduce the cost of their medical care.

Mental Illness As a Phospholipid Spectrum Disorder

"On the physical level, what you have with every mental illness is a phospholipid spectrum disorder," states Dr. Weeks, crediting Dr. David Horrobin and his landmark book *Phospholipid Spectrum Disorder in Psychiatry* (Marius Press, 1999) as the source of this concept that has the potential to produce radical change in the psychiatric field.

As discussed previously, deficiency in essential fatty acids can be a factor in mood disorders. While research has established this link, very few scientists or healing professionals are investigating the relationship between oils and light and the issue of light metabolism. (Oils as a category includes fats and essential fatty acids. Light metabolism refers to how the substance of light is handled in the body.) Here, Dr. Weeks explains the relationship and its significance for mental well-being:

> "At the biochemical level, cell membrane abnormalities (phospholipid disturbance) are directly implicated in mental illness. But what does that mean in terms of light metabolism? What have oils to do with light? What have light and oil to do with mood disorders? These questions can be understood on the biochemical level as well as on the metaphysical level.
>
> "*Phos* is Greek for 'light,' and *lipid* means 'oil,' so one could restate the word *phospholipid* as 'lighted oil.' The ancients taught 'All life from light,' yet today we smear on sunscreen immoderately and hide from the source of our life. Balance in light exposure is critically important. Disruptions in light metabolism contribute to sleep disruption, for example, which itself directly contributes to mental illnesses, most notably mania and depression.
>
> "What about the role of oil in mental illness? Oil has served throughout our human development as a dependable source of light. Oil is the least terrestrial of our physical substances; its hydrogen is the 'lightest' of all elements and therefore has the least relationship to the

earth. Oils have always been used to anoint kings, not for comfort alone but also to enhance the king's ability to receive cosmic wisdom from heaven for the benefit of his subjects on Earth . . . Sixty percent of the brain's dry weight is oil. Thus the term 'fat and happy.'

"Yet American consumers are taught to be terrified of oils in their diet. Patients tell me that these low-fat diets 'drive me crazy.' I do not discourage my patients from eating organic fatty foods as long as they are also getting regular exercise and minding their cardiovascular health. The ubiquitous phospholipid membranes, literally our custom agents for all cell-to-cell communication, are built from a diet rich in essential fatty acids."

Dr. Weeks expresses the hope that in the future medical professionals will refer to a range of mental disorders simply as phospholipid spectrum disorder, rather than labeling them bipolar disorder, major depressive disorder, or another psychiatric term. And as an accompanying revolution in treatment, "omega-3 fatty acids may represent a new class of membrane-active psychotropic compounds, and may herald the advent of a new class of rationally designed mood-stabilizing drugs."[171]

"Nobody Has a Prozac Deficiency"

In addition to the protocol of supplements and other measures taken on the physical level, Dr. Weeks encourages his patients with bipolar disorder to consider the effect of certain activities or environments on their mental/emotional states. For example, computer games and television have an "overhyping effect" on the brain. Highly stimulating environments may be problematic for them as well. Bipolar disorder can be regarded as a "kindling response," he observes. "Kindling is a neurological response. It suggests that when a cell has problems, it spreads it to the next cell, the next cell, the next cell, and so forth. With bipolar, there is a subseizure sort of process going. Kindling needs to be well controlled. This means that you've got to control stimulation to a certain degree."

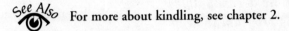 For more about kindling, see chapter 2.

In some cases, Dr. Weeks uses a low dose (5 mg daily) of lithium orotate, a form of natural lithium that does not create the problems associated with lithium carbonate, the form prescribed in conventional psychiatry, usually in dosages of 900 or 1200 mg daily.

"Very few people have frank lithium deficiencies," he says. "Nobody has a Prozac deficiency. No one has a Depakote or a Tegretol deficiency. While these medications help by suppressing the symptoms, they don't address the real issue, which is often addressed in a curative way by some of the things I'm talking about—the B vitamins, amino acids, and fish oil."

If someone comes to Dr. Weeks before starting on the drugs typically described for bipolar disorder, he is easily able with this program to keep them from having to start, he says. Further, the natural protocol has the advantage of not dulling the brilliance often associated with the condition. This dulling effect is one of the reasons noncompliance in taking medications is high among those with bipolar disorder.

Many of the people who come to Dr. Weeks have already been on drugs, however, as was the case with Derek, whose story follows. In these cases, the protocol is a complementary approach. It is not necessary, nor is it safe, to suddenly stop the medications. "By figuring out what you're deficient in and replenishing that, and what you're toxic in and diminishing that, gradually you need less and less medications, and ultimately get off them," explains Dr. Weeks.

"You can't simply stop the drugs," he says. If you do, "you can get a rebound problem or a detoxification problem. It's much easier if people can avoid the drugs at first, but the drugs are life-saving in many cases." Dr. Weeks stresses that while most of his patients are able to get off their drugs on this protocol, some of those "who came in on medications have to stay on medications to a certain degree."

If someone comes to Dr. Weeks before starting on the drugs typically described for bipolar disorder, he is easily able with this program to keep them from having to start, he says. Further, the natural protocol has the advantage of not dulling the brilliance often associated with the condition. This dulling effect is one of the reasons noncompliance in taking medications is high among those with bipolar disorder.

Dr. Weeks has found that for the most part with bipolar disorder he doesn't need to add homeopathic or anthroposophical medicine to the protocol. The physical measures prove sufficient. It is important to emphasize again, however, that treatment must be individualized.

"That comes back to the general homeopathic principle that everyone's earache is different. Everyone's spirit, astral, and etheric bodies have different relationships with each of the other members," says Dr. Weeks. The restoration of balance and harmony in body, mind, and spirit is an individual matter.

Mind and Spirit

One aspect of exploring the psychological dimension of disease is helping people to see that we are all in a position to determine what we think about, says Dr. Weeks. "People need to appreciate the fact that they're responsible for their reality. Their reality is entirely dependent upon their thought process." He emphasizes that this does not translate into blaming people for their illness. It is a matter of information and understanding. Once people see that they have a choice about what they think about, they can learn not to dwell on thoughts that increase their manic or depressed feelings. This psychotherapeutic model is known as Psychology of Mind, or the Health Realization model, and was developed in the 1970s by psychologists George S. Pransky, Ph.D., and Roger C. Mills, Ph.D., based on the ideas of Theosophist Sydney Banks.

 For information about Psychology of Mind, see the website www.psychologyofmind.com; or contact Pransky and Associates, P.O. Box 506, LaConner, WA 98257; tel: 360-466-5200.

Dr. Weeks also asks his patients what meaning their illness has for them, what purpose they think it serves. Generally, the first few times he asks them, they say they don't know. But on the third or fourth time, they have an answer. "Patients have been disempowered by doctors who don't ask for their participation," he notes, adding that many doctors ignore what patients say about why they are sick. The result is that "the patients have stopped informing the doctors."

With bipolar disorder, a common response to Dr. Weeks' question about purpose and meaning is, "I act this way because this is how I get my energy up to be creative. The reason I have this is because it keeps me in touch with my creativity." To that, Dr. Weeks responds, "Great, what a nice goal. Is there a more reasonable way for you to achieve that same goal?" When it comes to the depression pole in bipolar, some view it as the necessary rest period after going "a million miles an hour," he says, observing that "it's hard for people to attribute meaning to the depression because it is so painful."

When it comes to the spiritual realm, Dr. Weeks believes "that the spirit informs the soul, the soul informs the vitality, the life forces, and the life forces inform the physical body, more so than vice versa. I think we're fundamentally spiritual beings trying to make the world a better place, and basically learning how to love. To focus on the material is to miss the game."

He explains to his patients that spirit requires that they figure out what they want to do with their life. He asks them, "Why are you alive? How are you going to mean something with your life? Who are you going to help?" These are spiritual questions and not having answered them can be a component of mental illness, says Dr. Weeks. "Maybe a deficiency of doing something valuable in their own eyes, not in my judgmental eyes, but in *their* eyes, contributed to their illness."

Dr. Weeks is in agreement with Dr. Klinghardt (chapter 3) that healing happens faster from the spiritual level downward. "Whether it's homeopathy or talk therapy or something else, we can affect the physical body more from the top down than from the bottom up," he says. This is not license to neglect treatment at the physical level, however. "To simply do the top down, and ignore the fact that the person has an essential fatty acid deficiency, you're stepping on the gas and the brake," he says. His approach is to take care of the various factors concurrently.

Derek: Off the Drugs

When Derek came to Dr. Weeks, he was on lithium and trazodone (antidepressant), Depakote (anticonvulsant), Halcion (sleeping pill), and the tranquilizer clonazepam as needed. At 44, he had been struggling with bipolar disorder for 25 years. It wasn't his idea to consult another doctor, however. He had come to please his older brother. He was quite manic at the first appointment—"grandiose, hypersexual, expansive, pressured speech, typical manic process," recalls Dr. Weeks.

Derek sat sipping a Coke he had brought with him while Dr. Weeks introduced the notion that moods change with food. Derek agreed with the concept, reporting that chocolate and ice cream made him feel good. Dr. Weeks then explained the hypoglycemia process, using the illustration of how coffee and doughnuts make you feel good for a while, and then you crash. He gave Derek some articles to read on the subject.

Next, Dr. Weeks talked about sleep and exercise, how important it was for people with bipolar disorder to make sure that they get a good night's sleep and to exercise regularly, to get a rhythm going in their lives. "He was enjoying all this," said Dr. Weeks, "but he had no intention of giving up Coke or making any other changes." Derek submitted to a blood test before leaving.

At his next appointment three weeks later, he was still in his manic state and had acted on none of Dr. Weeks' suggestions. "I sat him down and showed him his blood results, which revealed all sorts of severe deficiencies. Now I had his attention, because I kind of popped his bubble, where he thought he was grandiose and perfect." He was deficient in all the essential fatty acids and neurotransmitter amino acids, and had severe intestinal dysbiosis, with candidiasis and the attendant buildup of toxins in the body.

Dr. Weeks recommended the appropriate supplements to redress his deficiencies and also gave him a natural sleep aid. In addition, he talked about dietary changes, specifically the avoidance of foods that feed the *Candida* yeast (see chapter 2), to help restore intestinal health. In the month that followed, Derek was noncompliant and disregarded the treatment. But at the end of the month he was back because he had plunged into depression. At that point, he was ready to listen. "When you're in a depression, you want to get out of it. You can take direction then," says Dr. Weeks.

He gave Derek vitamin B injections and essential fatty acid supplements. Within two weeks, his depression, which normally lasted for several months, had lifted, and he did not go into a manic phase, which was also his pattern. (He was a rapid cycler, going up and down every two to three months.) With that development, Dr. Weeks had Derek's attention. He took the EFAs religiously and gave himself vitamin B shots, according to the doctor's instructions. He took tryptophan to help him sleep, and GHB in a very low dose if he started to feel himself getting manic. GHB (gamma-hydroxybutyric acid), a carbohydrate naturally present in the human body, is synthesized from and converted back into GABA; dietary sources of GHB are animal and many vegetable proteins.[173]

Derek also implemented the recommended dietary changes, ate a nutritious diet rather than junk food, gave up Coke and other detrimental beverages, drank lots of water with a little lemon instead, and made sure he got exercise. The dietary changes were sufficient in his case to restore his intestinal balance.

After a month of compliance with this program, Derek was off all of his prescription drugs. "A typical taper schedule lasts from one to three months depending upon the degree of compliance," states Dr. Weeks. Now, three years later, Derek has still not had a bipolar episode. He continues to take the EFAs and maintain good eating and exercise habits.

As for the psychospiritual component of his disorder, "he didn't really discover the message, but he discovered that there *was* a message, and part of his life process is to figure that out," says Dr. Weeks. He did develop a sense of appreciation for the quieter joys in life, however, instead of running after manic highs. Perhaps you could say that he developed "a more mature sense of appreciation." His relationship with his wife improved tremendously and his children have a father for the first time.

For the process of cultivating this appreciation, the psychology of mind approach was very important, says Dr. Weeks. Derek learned that he chose to think that the manic highs are more fun and he can now choose to think that spending time with his children is the real fun, and far more satisfying. He knows now that it's up to him what he thinks, and he can control it. As for his creativity, Derek does not feel that it was cut off with the end of the manic episodes. He just views his process differently now.

In conclusion, Dr. Weeks notes that many people have the biochemical deficiencies and toxicities that testing of Derek's cellular terrain revealed, and they don't develop psychiatric components. In his view, the difference lies in the realm of soul and spirit, and it is up to the individuals involved to explore that mystery if they want to get to the other facets of their bipolar disorder.

5 Biochemical Treatment of Bipolar Disorder

Biochemical researcher William J. Walsh, Ph.D., chief scientist at the Health Research Institute and Pfeiffer Treatment Center (HRI-PTC), is the heir-apparent of the late Carl Pfeiffer, M.D., Ph.D., a pioneer in the biochemical treatment of illness, and of mental illnesses in particular. Before he died, Dr. Pfeiffer asked Dr. Walsh to establish the center to carry on the important work in which they had both been engaged for decades.

HRI-PTC is a not-for-profit research and outpatient facility near Chicago, in Warrenville, Illinois. HRI is the research wing and PTC the treatment wing. Designed as a collaboration between biochemists and medical doctors, the organization specializes in biochemical treatment of mental, emotional, and behavioral disorders. Since its founding in 1989, it has treated more than 15,000 people with bipolar disorder, depression and anxiety disorders, schizophrenia, autism, attention deficit disorder, hyperactivity, and other behavioral, emotional, and learning problems.

"What I've been doing for the last 25 or 30 years," explains Dr. Walsh, "is trying to develop chemical classifications for conditions such as bipolar disorder, depression, schizophrenia, behavior disorders, and autism because every one of these terms is an umbrella term or a garbage term that encompasses different categories." The chemistry underlying the diagnosis is not only the key to individual treatment, but if biochemical commonalities could be found among

What Is Biochemical Treatment?

Biochemical treatment is the supplemental use of substances that naturally occur in the body (for example, vitamins, minerals, amino acids, and enzymes) to rebalance an individual's disturbed biochemistry. The therapy operates on the tenet of biochemical individuality, which holds that every individual's biochemistry is unique and treatment must identify and address the unique condition. Treatment also considers the effects of environmental and food supply toxins, and includes natural detoxification protocols as needed.

individuals in each category, this could also potentially point the way to the cause of the disorder, with attendant prevention and even cure.

Although bipolar disorder clearly has a genetic component, that doesn't mean that the condition is "hopeless or incurable," says Dr. Walsh. "What genetics means, to me, is chemistry. Chemistry can be adjusted and corrected." He gives the example of someone with depression, in which a genetic component is involved (science acknowledges the role of genetics in depression). "Some people, whether with medication or with some other therapy, become free of depression. So does that mean it wasn't genetic? And they weren't really depressed?"

About two-thirds of the bipolar patients who come to PTC have "classical" bipolar disorder while one-third are bipolar with psychotic features, Dr. Walsh reports. "Bipolar with psychotic features may just be a more severe version of bipolar," he says, noting that all illness occurs as mild, moderate, or severe. "If you have a mild version, you'll be hypomanic. If it's moderate, you might be a classic manic-depressive. If it's severe, then you might have bipolar with psychotic features."

Some patients with hypomania rather than full-blown manic episodes "still feel that it's out of control, that it's wrecking their life. They can't trust themselves," notes Dr. Walsh. Others, experiencing their hypomanic periods as their most creative time, "want to get rid of the depression and keep the mania. But the severe manic-depressives, they want to get rid of both."

Symptomatically and biochemically, bipolar with psychotic features is close to schizophrenia, states Dr. Walsh. "I've seen almost identical patients with identical symptoms and one is called schizophrenic and the other is called bipolar with psychotic features. I think it's just a matter of semantics." In addition, the blood and urine tests of people with the two conditions show the same results. "We can't tell the difference between the biochemistry of the schizophrenic and the bipolar with psychotic features." Dr. Walsh notes that this is not the case with classical bipolar.

In biochemical treatment, it is the details of the biochemistry rather than the diagnostic labels that provide the direction for therapy. This approach has the advantage of addressing each person's unique biochemical condition. In contrast to prescription drugs designed to elevate serotonin or lower dopamine, biochemical therapy gives the body only what it needs, and it does so safely. The problem with the pharmaceuticals is that they're "affecting probably five to 15 other neurotransmitters, altering these people's brains and causing these things called side effects," says Dr. Walsh.

Providing the body with missing nutrients restores its innate ability to correct and regulate its neurotransmitter levels and function. "It seems likely that the next century's treatments will implement natural body chemicals that restore the patient to a normal condition, rather than drugs that result in an abnormal condition," Dr. Walsh states. "The world may eventually learn the wisdom of Pfeiffer's Law: For every drug that benefits a patient, there is a natural substance that can achieve the same effect."[174]

Biochemical Features of Bipolar Disorder

While every individual is different, the top four biochemical trends in frequency of occurrence in the people with bipolar disorder who come to PTC are a methylation disorder that results in too high or too low levels of neurotransmitters, essential fatty acid imbalance, metal metabolism problems, and pyroluria, a disorder that leads to extreme deficiencies in zinc, vitamin B_6, and arachidonic acid, an omega-6 essential fatty acid.

These imbalances may be mild, moderate, or severe, which has a bearing on whether a person develops bipolar disorder or not. On the mild end of the spectrum, "if a person is in a great environment and life is pretty copacetic and calm, they may go through life without a breakdown," states Dr. Walsh. However, if a person on the mild end "has a nasty environment or some troubling traumatic events in their life, they might break down because of that. But at the other end of the spectrum, with severe versions of these imbalances, I think it's inevitable. It doesn't matter what their life circumstances are, it's going to happen."

Methylation Problem

In the 1970s, Dr. Pfeiffer developed a biochemical treatment model for schizophrenia that forms the foundation for the approach PTC uses today with both schizophrenia and bipolar disorder. Dr. Pfeiffer's model was based on his discovery of high histamine levels in some schizophrenics. Others had low histamine levels. Histamine is an essential protein metabolite (a product of metabolism) found in all body tissues, and although most people associate it with allergies (it is what produces the runny nose, weepy eyes, and other signs of inflammation in an allergic reaction), in the brain, histamine functions as a neurotransmitter.

Dr. Pfeiffer found that he could reverse or alleviate schizophrenic symptoms by giving supplements that normalized the histamine level, lowering or raising it as needed. He concluded from the effectiveness of this approach that histamine, as a neurotransmitter, might very well be the decisive factor in schizophrenia, recalls Dr. Walsh. "A lot of time has passed since his death, and there's a lot more evidence. It appears that histamine is actually a marker for methylation. People who are high histamine are undermethylated. People who are low histamine are overmethylated. What Pfeiffer did was accidentally stumble on the right treatment, on an effective treatment. He thought he was adjusting histamine, but what he was doing was adjusting the methyl-folate ratio."

What do *undermethylation* and *overmethylation* mean? Methyl is one of the more common organic chemicals in the body; methyl groups are present in most enzymes and proteins. Methylation is the process by which methyl groups are added to a compound, making methyl available for the many reactions for which it is needed in the body. Both methyl and histamine are major, ubiquitous chemicals in the body, and they compete with each other, Dr. Walsh explains.

With too much methyl, the body overproduces the three neurotransmitters dopamine, norepinephrine, and serotonin. With too little methyl, the neurotransmitter levels are too low. Folates are the various forms that folic acid takes in the body. Folic acid, a member of the B-vitamin family, aids in the manufacture of brain neurotransmitters and thus needs to be available in the proper ratio with methyl.

On the basis of his research since the 1970s, Dr. Walsh now

> On the basis of his research since the 1970s, Dr. Walsh now knows that the methylation factor operates not only in schizophrenia but in bipolar and other mental disorders as well. . . . As with schizophrenia, most people with bipolar disorder have a methyl imbalance—too much or too little.

knows that the methylation factor operates not only in schizophrenia but in bipolar and other mental disorders as well. For example, high histamine and its attendant low methyl are also associated with obsessive-compulsive disorders. As with schizophrenia, most people with bipolar disorder have a methyl imbalance—either too much or too little. "The methylation factor highlights the importance of knowing what is happening in a person biochemically," observes Dr. Walsh. "For people who are overmethylated, taking drugs to raise neurotransmitter levels will be detrimental."

Treatment for low histamine and overmethylation consists of supplements to reduce methyl, notably folic acid, vitamin B_{12}, and vitamin B_3 (niacin or niacinamide). Many people in this category also have a metal metabolism problem, as evidenced by high levels

The High-Histamine Personality

"What histamine does is it speeds up the body's metabolism," states Patrick Holford, founder of the Institute for Optimum Nutrition in London, England. "It 'turns up the fire.' [High-histamine people] tend to be compulsive and obsessive in their personality. They wake up early and their mind is always thinking. This is not a problem. There are an awful lot of very successful people, creative people, multimillionaires, and so on, and they are high-histamine people. They're kind of driven people. However, the high-histamine people tend to become deficient in nutrients because they burn nutrients faster. So if they're on a bad diet, that sort of obsessive tendency can flip over into mental illness."[175]

of copper in relationship to low zinc, so that problem needs to be addressed as well (see the section on metal metabolism to follow).

The supplements used in treating high histamine and undermethylation are the amino acid methionine, calcium, magnesium, and vitamin B_6. These supplements increase methyl in the body and/or assist in methylation. Calcium is an important supplement for those who are undermethylated because it helps lower histamine levels. For those people who do not efficiently convert methionine to SAMe (S-adenosyl methionine), a necessary step in making methyl available to the body, SAMe supplements are part of their program.

With this protocol, "neurotransmitter production will become more normal," Dr. Walsh explains. However, reversing undermethylation is "a slow, gradual process that takes four to six months to complete."

In addition, the nature of high-histamine, undermethylated people sometimes interferes with treatment. It is important to note here that this biochemical characteristic exists not only among people with bipolar disorder or other "mental" illness, but widely in the general population as well. Those who manifest bipolar have a more severe imbalance, genetic vulnerability, or other factors that combine to produce the disorder. "High-histamine, undermethylated people are intrinsically noncompliant," says Dr. Walsh. "High-histamine, undermethylated people are the kind of people who don't want to go see a doctor for anything. If they have a splitting headache, they won't even take an aspirin. They tend to be averse to treatment of any kind."

While the supplements to correct these biochemical trends tend to be the same, there is no standard protocol at the Pfeiffer Treatment Center. Treatment is based on individual biochemistry and dosage is determined according to a person's metabolic weight factor. This is a method of calculating dosages based on metabolism, Dr. Walsh explains. It is far more accurate than figuring dosage as a mere percentage of the standard 160-pound person. The latter method results in underdosing small people and overdosing big people. If you have someone who is 320 pounds, for example, it is not correct to give them twice the dose of a 160-pound person, says Dr. Walsh.

Essential Fatty Acid Imbalance

In Dr. Walsh's experience, essential fatty acid (EFA) imbalances play a much greater role in bipolar disorder than they do in either unipolar depression or schizophrenia. "That might be the differentiating factor between them," he notes. "Of the 300 major fats in neuronal tissue and the myelin sheath, four of them make up more than 90 percent of all this fatty material at brain synapses and receptors. That has to be important." The four fatty acids are EPA (eicosapentaenoic acid), DHA (docosahexaenoic acid), AA (arachidonic acid), and DGLA (dihomo-gamma-linolenic acid). The first two are omega-3 essential fatty acids and the second two are omega-6s.

As others have observed, the standard American diet, with its generally poor nutrition and emphasis on junk food, tends to result in an overload of omega-6 and a deficit of omega-3 EFAs, notes Dr. Walsh. Both the low- and high-histamine categories of bipolar disorder fit this profile. The main EFA therapy for these people is omega-3 supplementation, specifically EPA and DHA. Fish oil contains both, and is therefore a helpful form of supplement, but Dr. Walsh also uses products that are pure EPA and

DHA. For bipolar, he does not use flax oil as a source of omega 3s because, being primarily EPA, it does not supply enough DHA.

With pyroluria (see section in this chapter), the problem is not omega-3 deficiency, but rather, low levels of omega 6, specifically, arachidonic acid. This is less common in bipolar disorder than the methyl factor. In these cases, the EFA supplement needed is primrose oil or borage oil. Dr. Walsh observes that people with bipolar disorder and this biochemistry have the typical skin problems associated with omega-6 deficiency, which are very dry skin, inability to tan, and vulnerability to sun poisoning.

With people who demonstrate the omega-3 deficiency, a fascinating fact is that DHA and EPA address the opposing poles of bipolar disorder. DHA works to calm the manic phase and EPA helps to lift the depressive phase, says Dr. Walsh. Taken together, they act as a mood regulatory system and help prevent mood swings. Both are needed, which is a further explanation of why fish oil, which contains both, produces results in treating bipolar disorder, while flax oil does not, as research shows.

Hypothetically, says Dr. Walsh, people who only experience mild hypomania rather than full-blown mania in their bipolar disorder and who want to avoid only the depressive phase could take EPA alone, but he typically recommends the combination of the two essential fatty acids.

Metal Metabolism Problem

A problem with metal metabolism (the regulation of metals, which include both necessary minerals and toxic heavy metals such as mercury) in the body is also frequently present in bipolar disorder, as evidenced by high levels of copper in relation to zinc. This indicates that the body is unable to control the mineral levels in the bloodstream. Normally, the body can maintain homeostasis (the proper ratio) of copper and zinc in the blood, regardless of diet or other factors, because this ratio is so crucial to many functions. This mechanism of homeostasis relies upon a vital protein called metallothionein; thus, an inability to maintain homeostasis indicates a metallothionein deficiency or malfunction.

Metallothionein is involved in many functions of the body, including immunity, brain and gastrointestinal tract maturation, and the regulation of metals. A deficiency in or inability to utilize this substance is associated with an impaired nervous system; mental difficulties; weakened immunity; and digestive problems including malabsorption, nutritional deficiencies, and the development of allergies. Dr. Walsh has also discovered a link between autism and metallothionein dysfunction; in fact, his research suggests that such dysfunction may be a primary cause of autism.

 For more about the autism-metallothionein link and Dr. Walsh's work, see the author's *The Natural Medicine Guide to Autism* (Hampton Roads, 2002).

Since there is no commercial test to measure metallothionein in the body, PTC relies on the ratio of blood levels of zinc, copper, and ceruloplasmin (a substance in the blood to which copper attaches) as indicators of malfunction of this protein. Treatment then consists of supplements to stimulate the function of metallothionein.

PTC has long been expert at correcting disturbances in metal metabolism. "We've known for more than 25 years that two-thirds of people with behavior disorders have a metal metabolism problem," states Dr. Walsh. "And we've known for all that time that it was almost certainly a problem with metallothionein. The reason we were sure was because all of the metals that are managed by metallothionein are the very ones that are abnormal in these people."

For example, people with obsessive-compulsive disorder tend to have very low copper levels, he explains, as do sociopaths (people with antisocial personality disorder). In bipolar disorder, the undermethylated type also has low copper, while the overmethylated type has high copper levels, and the pyroluric type has severe zinc and metallothionein deficiencies. Dr. Walsh emphasizes that it is the ratio of copper to zinc that is important here. "We learned a while ago that you have to measure the ratio to get solid data. If you look at the individual elements, you can get fooled."

A metallothionein problem, which results in a failure to achieve homeostasis of copper and zinc in the bloodstream, is mainly a genetic disorder, according to Dr. Walsh. But a zinc deficiency can also create or further exacerbate the problem. "The primary nutrient needed in the formation of metallothionein is zinc, so if you're extraordinarily zinc deficient, that will disable the system," says Dr. Walsh.

In any case, biochemical treatment is the solution to reversing the problem. "Zinc, manganese, and vitamins E and C are all aimed at inducing and promoting normal functioning of metallothionein," explains Dr. Walsh, adding that selenium and glutathione (a relative of glutamic acid, an amino acid) are also very useful nutrients for this purpose. Vitamin B_6 is also part of the protocol because "B_6 and zinc work together, and B_6 is directly involved in the synthesis of some of the neurotransmitters."

Dr. Walsh has found this program to be "quite effective." Typically, the copper and zinc level out and become normalized. "When the person achieves homeostasis of copper and zinc levels in the blood, you can conclude that metallothionein is operational," he says.

As the supplement program gradually brings the metallothionein protein into proper function, metallothionein's detoxification work will resume. The emphasis here is on *gradual*. "We learned long ago that we don't dare suddenly bring it to life," Dr. Walsh explains. "Because if that happens, the metallothionein works so well that it suddenly causes an excessive amount of toxics in the tissues to be released all at once. And that could cause nasty symptoms and stress the kidneys." To prevent this, the dosages of the supplements that stimulate metallothionein are slowly increased over time.

Pyroluria

In some cases of bipolar disorder, tests reveal a condition called pyroluria, which is characterized by extreme deficiencies in zinc, vitamin B_6, and arachidonic acid, the omega-6 essential fatty acid discussed above.

A pyrrole is a basic chemical structure used in the manufacture of heme, which is what makes the blood red. Pyroluria is a genetic disorder in pyrrole chemistry, characterized by an overproduction of kryptopyrroles (meaning "hidden pyrroles") during the synthesis of hemoglobin (the iron-rich component of the blood that carries oxygen). Since kryptopyrroles bind with vitamin B_6 and zinc, which are then excreted in the urine, this leads to deficiencies in these two nutrients. People with pyroluria may have low levels of the neurotransmitter serotonin, as vitamin B_6 is needed for its synthesis.[176] Also, GABA is a zinc-dependent neurotransmitter, so a zinc deficiency may have negative repercussions on this neurotransmitter as well.

Pyroluria is known to scientists and physicians with a biochemical orientation for its connection to schizophrenia, says Dr. Walsh, but bipolar disorder is associated with it as well, and the two diagnostic labels are often confused when pyroluria is present. Pyroluria is a genetic disorder that may explode into mental imbalance as a result of a stressful event or period in one's life. "With the pyrolurics, not only do they have a high-stress onset, but their relapses almost always are tied to stress. It's a cause and effect there, whereas with the other two groups [classic bipolar disorder and schizophrenia], it's not necessarily related to their life circumstances. They cycle also, but there's no rationale to it."

The involvement of pyroluria in bipolar disorder and schizophrenia is consistent with the first breakdown typically taking place between the ages of 15 and 25. Dr. Walsh believes that puberty and the growth spurt of that time period exacerbate the pyroluria by consuming zinc and elevating copper, and serve to trigger the mental disorders. "Hormones are related to copper," he explains. "The higher your estrogen level, the higher your copper level. Copper is related to paranoid schizophrenia, so that's a direct connection. Also, for the pyrolurics, zinc deficiency is a problem. When you go through a growth spurt, it consumes a lot of zinc, so a pyroluric under a growth spurt may become severely zinc deficient."

The classic signs of zinc and B_6 deficiency, which tend to go together, serve as an alert for pyroluria. These include sensitivity to bright light, little or no dream recall, a tendency to skip breakfast, and preference for spicy food. Treatment for pyroluria focuses on supplementation with zinc, vitamin B$_6$, and augmenting nutrients.

Correcting Biochemical Imbalances

As part of gathering information for treatment design, PTC looks "for the symptoms that tend to accompany the various biochemical imbalances that our work over decades has taught us are associated with these disorders, and then we do a history that takes an hour to an hour and a half," says Dr. Walsh. "We want to learn everything about that human being. We want to know their medical history, their symptoms, their personality, their life history, the kind of student they were, reaction to any medications they had. We want to know what happened at the time of their breakdown. We want to know what differences they felt and their family saw at the time of the breakdown."

The scientific basis for biochemical treatment, however, is gained from blood and urine tests. Blood testing is the key for high and low histamine, or undermethylation and overmethylation, respectively. In the case of pyroluria, it is a urine test. With this information, treatment can be tailored to the individual.

 In addition to the Pfeiffer Treatment Center (see the listing for Dr. Walsh in the appendix), another clinic that specializes in this type of biochemical balancing is the Olive Garvey Center for Healing Arts, Center for the Improvement of Human Functioning International, 3100 North Hillside, Wichita, KS 67219; tel: (316) 682-3100; website: www.brightspot.org.

PTC has had good success with bipolar disorder in most cases, based on outcome studies, with most families reporting "remarkable improvement" or "partial improvement." No improvement is uncommon with the biochemical approach, reports Dr. Walsh. Those who experience partial improvement can be divided into two categories: "those who did great and relapse once in a while; and those who got partially better and are still partially better."

Partial improvement suggests to him that the chemistry is only partially corrected. "There is still some element of chemical imbalance present and all it takes is an environmental trigger—it could be an emotional upset, a death in the family, an illness, an injury, a car accident," he says. The relapses are almost never back to the pretreatment state, however. He describes it as going from zero to 100 percent with treatment and then with relapse going down to 60 percent. Relapse seems to be a combination of stress and compliance problems, reports Dr. Walsh. The relapses are usually brief and, with resumed or temporarily increased dosage of supplements, the person is soon back up to 100 percent.

> PTC *has had good success with bipolar disorder in most cases, based on outcome studies, with most families reporting "remarkable improvement" or "partial improvement." No improvement is uncommon with the biochemical approach, reports Dr. Walsh.*

"We strike out 20 to 25 percent of the time in bipolar," he says, citing compliance among older patients as a major issue. "We've done outcome studies of thousands of people and we find that compliance is almost linearly heading downward from the age of three. So the older the person, the less likely they are to comply with your treatment."

People with bipolar disorder are different from schizophrenics in this regard. The latter seem be more compliant perhaps because "they suffer so dramatically," says Dr. Walsh. "Their pain is so enormous that they will do anything to get better. I think it's a matter of desperation for them." This is not to say that people with bipolar disorder are not suffering extremely, but schizophrenics are further along the continuum of pain and dysfunction in life.

One of the reasons for noncompliance may be negative experiences with medications. By the time most of the people who are

In Their Own Words

"It took me far too long to realize that lost years and relationships cannot be recovered, that damage done to oneself and others cannot always be put right again, and that freedom from the control imposed by medication loses its meaning when the only alternatives are death and insanity."[177]

—Kay Redfield Jamison, Ph.D.

bipolar come to PTC, they have been on many medications and suffered through their negative effects. In a not uncommon occurrence, one young man recently told Dr. Walsh that he didn't think he could bear to live if he had to continue to take Zyprexa (an atypical antipsychotic) and Celexa (an SSRI). He was on a high dose of both and didn't think they were helping him. "He said he felt like he was a horse with blinders on and he could only see straight ahead when he was thinking about things," recalls Dr. Walsh. "It was an interesting way to describe the differences in his mental functioning. He would try to focus on something and would lose all perspective."

For many people, the effects associated with the drugs they have been given in an attempt to regulate their bipolar disorder have left them with an aversion to medication. "We give them capsules to swallow and it's hard for them to distinguish between medication and nutrient therapy," observes Dr. Walsh, who views gaining compliance as a component of a successful therapeutic method. "You need to have a treatment that people can do and will do. That's part of the treatment."

If people stop taking the supplements for a while, even a week or ten days, they begin to deteriorate. Then they are even less likely to take their supplements. "Sometimes it's a vicious circle. Once you get to a certain point, then you're not able to bring yourself back. It can happen quickly."

Patients with bipolar disorder have to take more supplements than most PTC patients, an average of seven to ten pills, both morning and evening. Compounding the supplements (a compounding pharmacy prepares the formula in accordance with the individual's biochemical needs) makes compliance more likely, as it usually cuts the number of pills down to three to four, taken twice daily.

The following cases feature the two types of methylation problems in bipolar disorder and the efficacy of biochemical therapy in reversing the condition.

Elena: Low-Histamine, Overmethylated Bipolar

Elena, 24, had always been an excellent student and high achiever; she was valedictorian of her high school class and graduated summa cum laude from a prestigious university. After college, she went to law school. In her first year, she had a severe breakdown, was diagnosed with bipolar disorder, and had to go back home to her family. When her parents brought her to PTC, Elena had been sick for a year. She was on medication and undergoing counseling, but had cut off contact with all of her friends, was no longer able to work, and rarely left her bedroom.

"We found that she was one of the lowest histamine people we had ever seen," Dr. Walsh reports. "That seemed to be her only imbalance. Everything else was normal and because this wasn't completely consistent with her symptoms, we retested her and verified that in fact that was her proper diagnosis." Her overmethylated state meant that "she had too much dopamine, norepinephrine, and serotonin, which explained why the SSRI she was taking was a failure." The drug was prescribed to try and enhance serotonin activity, "but she was a person who already had too much serotonin."

To address Elena's overmethylation, the Pfeiffer Center gave her folic acid, vitamin B_{12}, and niacinamide with augmenting nutrients, including vitamins C, E, and B_6. The B_{12} was delivered in the form of weekly injections. In the beginning, she wasn't well enough to give herself these injections, but when she had improved, PTC taught her how to do them herself, and thereafter she did. With such low histamine, she had to continue the shots.

Elena "responded marvelously" to this simple program. In the second month on it, she began to improve and by the fourth month was back to normal. Dr. Walsh notes that essential fatty acids were not part of her regimen because this was before the connection between essential fatty acids and bipolar disorder was known. Today, Elena is doing fine, has not had a relapse, and is working as an attorney, having earned her law degree in the interim.

In fact, she returned to law school after the fourth month of treatment, believing that she was cured. "She completely violated my recommendations," recalls Dr. Walsh. "I wanted her to wait until at least eight months. She was just in a hurry to get on with her life and went back and struggled for a while. She put too much stress on herself during the biochemical transition period, before we had her chemistry completely fixed."

Dr. Walsh always cautions people, when they start feeling better, not to be in too big of a rush to get on with their lives. "Most of these people have lost a few years and they can't wait to get back. They feel behind. All their friends have graduated, are working, married . . . We always urge them not to jump into the deep end of the pool, but just to dip their toe in. We suggest that, instead of going through a difficult full set of college courses during the first year of recovery, they take one or two fairly easy courses and test out their brain and test out their ability to handle stress." Elena ignored this advice, went back into a difficult, full-time course of study, and "toughed her way through it." Fortunately, putting herself through tremendous stress did not have lasting repercussions on her condition.

Marcus: High-Histamine, Undermethylated Bipolar

Marcus was strikingly handsome—he looked like a movie star— and had a compelling personality. He had been diagnosed with classical bipolar disorder at 17 and when Dr. Walsh saw him at the age of 20, he had just spent a year in a penitentiary for forging his father's signature on checks during the excessive buying of a manic phase. His father was wealthy and had for a time paid the debts his son ran up on his manic shopping sprees. At some point, however, he cut his son off financially, thinking that he was enabling this behavior. Not long after, Marcus forged the checks and wound up in jail.

After his release from prison, his parents brought him to PTC. He had at various times been on the mood stabilizers lithium, Depakote, and Tegretol, but he didn't like any of them. While his parents thought the drugs helped, he said that they did not and refused to take them. On the other hand, "he seemed very interested in our treatment," says Dr. Walsh.

Testing revealed that "he was one of the undermethylated bipolars, with very high histamine." For this, the Pfeiffer doctors put him on the classic methylation program, that is, methionine, calcium, magnesium, zinc, vitamin B_6, manganese, and vitamins C and E.

Marcus complied with the protocol and in three months he was doing marvelously well. "Then at his six-month follow-up visit, he straggled in, looking sad. I asked him what had happened and he said, 'Well, I want to apologize. I stopped your program. Things were going so well I didn't think I needed all those capsules. I thought I could do it myself.'"

The result was relapse. He was plunged into a manic phase again, during which he bought two boats on false credit and was arrested a second time. He needed a lawyer, and his family had refused to help unless he came back to PTC.

Retesting revealed that his chemistry was as skewed as it had been before he started treatment. Marcus' program was adjusted slightly according to these results, but it was essentially the same regimen.

Marcus was sent back to prison for a second year. When he was about to be released at the end of that time, his mother called Dr. Walsh and told him that Marcus wanted to come to PTC. They drove there directly from the prison. Marcus told Dr. Walsh that he was never going to go through that again, meaning incarceration, and he vowed that he would be compliant. That was six years ago, and he is doing "remarkably well," by his own and his family's report. He has had no more major episodes, has established a successful career in business, and, as far as Dr. Walsh knows, has stuck to his vow to be compliant.

6 Amino Acids: Giving the Brain What It Needs

Julia Ross, M.A., who holds a master's degree in clinical psychology, is a pioneer in nutritional psychology and has 25 years of experience directing counseling programs that address mood problems, addiction, and eating disorders. Nutritional psychology recognizes the central role that biochemistry plays in mental health and regards nutritional intervention in the form of diet and supplements as an essential treatment for restoring that health.

Having witnessed the potent effects that amino acids and other nutrients can have on psychological states, in 1988 Ross established Recovery Systems, a clinic in Mill Valley, California, devoted to treating mood disorders, addiction, and eating disorders from a nutritional psychology orientation. Ross is director of the clinic and has detailed her approach in two books, *The Diet Cure* and *The Mood Cure*.

Amino acids (nutrients found in high-protein foods) are central to her work because they are the building blocks for neurotransmitters, those "unbelievably powerful natural mood stabilizers," as Ross describes them. The four neurotransmitters that feature consistently in the disorders Ross treats are serotonin, dopamine/norepinephrine, GABA, and endorphins. She combines dopamine and norepinephrine because the symptoms of deficiency are the same for both, as are the amino acids required for their synthesis. By giving the body the amino acid building blocks (in simple supplement form) for "whatever mood-enhancing neurotransmitters you have in short supply, they can typically be replenished quickly, easily, and safely," she states.[178]

See Also   **For more about amino acids, see chapter 2.**

In the case of bipolar disorder, L-tryptophan (or its converted form, 5-HTP) is the amino acid precursor most often required, says Ross, as the primary neurotransmitter deficiency involved is usually serotonin. L-tyrosine and L-phenylalanine can also be important, as they are the precursors to norepinephrine and dopamine, which are also implicated.

Ross recommends other amino acids as needed, based on the signs and symptoms the individual is manifesting, notably GABA, taurine, and glycine for calming; DL-phenylalanine for excessive emotional sensitivity; and L-glutamine to stabilize brain function by stabilizing blood sugar in the brain. If the person's diet has been chronically poor or other factors have resulted in overall amino acid depletion, a complete amino acid formula may also be indicated.[179]

The other components of Ross' treatment approach to bipolar disorder are omega-3 essential fatty acids in the form of fish oil, high-potency multivitamin/mineral supplements and a well-balanced diet to build a strong nutritional foundation, plus a recommendation to eliminate gluten-containing foods from the diet, which has proven beneficial for most of her bipolar clients.

Identifying Amino Acid Deficiencies

The first step in designing a treatment plan is to identify the individual's amino acid deficiencies. "You can't directly test the neurotransmitter levels in the brain," says Ross. "Testing blood levels of amino acids doesn't tell you exactly what's happening in the brain." Fortunately, the symptoms of deficiency of the neurotransmitters in question are "very obvious" and distinct from each other.

Ross gathers information about a client's full range of physical, emotional/psychological, and behavioral symptoms in an initial

In Their Own Words

After a highly publicized manic breakdown in 1996, during which she wandered, dazed and delusional, through the streets of Los Angeles until she was picked up by the police and taken to a psychiatric ward, actress Margot Kidder began to look for natural treatments for the bipolar disorder with which she had struggled for over two decades. Based on her research, she put together a protocol of amino acids, vitamins, and minerals, which she later learned are used by many orthomolecular physicians in treating people with bipolar disorder. (Orthomolecular medicine corrects [*ortho*] the molecular balance of the body, which means supplying the body with the amino acids, vitamins, minerals, and other substances it needs.)[180]

"Having spent over 20 years in and out of conventional Western psychiatrists' offices, being given almost every pill that they have in their arsenal and discovering that none of them really work, certainly not in the long term . . . ," Kidder states, "finally, after a last spectacular manic episode, I had really had enough and did a great deal of homework in alternate ways to balance out my system naturally rather than throwing synthetic drugs on top of symptoms. . . . And it's working—no symptoms, no ups, no downs, which in my life is nothing short of a miracle."[181]

Kidder has been free of symptoms for over five years and is now a strong advocate for patients' rights, speaking out about "the right to wellness" versus "pharmacological lobotomy, which is usually what you get."[182] The message of her own experience is "You *can* get better, contrary to what your psychiatrist may have told you. You can get better—and stay better."[183]

psychosocial assessment of that person and his or her family. A nutritional evaluation, medical workup, and basic blood work to determine vitamin and mineral status and blood sugar levels among other parameters are also part of the preliminaries to treatment recommendations.

Both serotonin and dopamine/norepinephrine deficiencies are characterized by depression, but the depressions are of different kinds. With low serotonin, it is the agitated, restless, anxious, worried form of depression, the negative, dark cloud variety, says Ross. "It is not the can't-get-out-of-bed kind. In fact, often they wish they could get *into* bed because they're up pacing and worrying, having dark thoughts at night." Suicidal thoughts and sleep problems of all kinds (inability to fall asleep, waking up in the night, inability to fall back asleep) are common, as are irritability, anger, and edginess. All forms of fear, from nervous worry to panic attacks, are also characteristic of serotonin deficiency.

While this cluster of symptoms may understandably cause people "to assume that they are seriously mentally ill, perhaps traumatized by an early childhood distress," notes Ross, having heard this from numerous clients, "in fact, in many cases all of it can be eliminated practically overnight by taking L-tryptophan or 5-HTP, which are quickly converted to serotonin."

In contrast to that of serotonin deficiency, the depression manifested in dopamine/norepinephrine deficiency is not an "agitated depression. This is the flat, wanting-to-stay-in-bed-all-day depression," explains Ross. With this neurotransmitter deficiency, people "are tired, they can't concentrate, and their vitality and ambition are compromised." L-tyrosine and L-phenylalanine are the amino acid supplements needed to reverse this deficiency. (Omega-3 fish oil is helpful with this kind of depression as well.)

A stressed-out, burned-out state is the number one symptom of GABA deficiency, says Ross. "People lacking in this neurotransmitter describe themselves as 'overwhelmed, stressed-out, burned-out, and tense.' They have that kind of wired inability to relax, but it's more physical than mental. They're stiff; their bodies tend to be erect rather than relaxed." They are chronically in the fight-or-flight response, with its attendant adrenaline flow. "They feel as if they're 'on' all the time, they can't turn it off, and they're exhausted from it." GABA as an amino acid supplement is indicated in these cases. The other "relaxing aminos" taurine and glycine can be used as corollary calming agents.

Endorphin deficiency can also be a factor, although neither GABA nor endorphin deficiency is endemic to bipolar disorder. Deficiencies in either may be present in depression of any kind, including that found in bipolar disorder. Deficiency of endorphins,

---

Symptoms of Neurotransmitter Deficiency or Dysfunction[185]

Serotonin
depression with negativity
low self-esteem
irritability, anger
anxiety, panic, phobias
obsessive thoughts/behaviors
suicidal ideation
sleep disturbances
heat intolerance
premenstrual syndrome

Endorphins
sensitivity to pain
emotional sensitivity
crying easily

Dopamine/Norepinephrine
depression with apathy
lack of energy
lack of drive
focus and concentration
  problems

GABA
inability to relax
stressed-out or burnt-out state
tight muscles

---

the natural painkillers, results in vulnerability to physical and emotional pain. Typical signs are being "overly sensitive to emotional injury. People hurt their feelings, and they just can't get over it," states Ross. "They're just emotionally exposed, raw." The amino acid building blocks for endorphins are DL-phenylalanine and D-phenylalanine.

L-glutamine is another amino acid that can be useful as general support and a source of fuel for the whole brain. Its primary role is to keep the blood sugar in the brain stable. The brain burns glutamine when it runs out of glucose in a hypoglycemic blood sugar drop, Ross explains. Supplementation with glutamine usually promotes "stable, calm, alert brain function."[184] It is typically needed when the person eats a lot of sweets and starches, has a high caffeine intake, and skips meals.

Feeding the Brain Its Natural Diet

The advantages of amino acid supplementation over prescription drugs aimed at neurotransmitter function are numerous. Unlike the drugs, which can take weeks to begin to work, supplementation produces effects rapidly, often in a matter of days or even hours, says Ross.

Also unlike drugs, amino acid supplementation addresses the underlying problems—that is, neurotransmitter deficiency and function—rather than manipulating brain chemistry in an unnatural way. And, as Dr. Walsh noted in the previous chapter, drugs may be designed to target certain neurotransmitters, but they alter the chemistry of the whole brain in the process. It is important to know that "people with bipolar tendencies can have negative as well as positive reactions to these amino acids," Ross states. The reactions subside, however, when the person stops taking the supplement.

Tryptophan has been the amino acid most often indicated for Ross' bipolar clients.

In Their Own Words

"[Lithium] stabilized me into a seething melancholy. . . . So I gradually pieced together from reading a lot of the papers from the Journal of Orthomolecular Medicine *which vitamins, minerals, and amino acids worked as teams and helped the brain restore normal function. And then of course I read a lot of things about diet. I didn't expect that would be a factor at all, but I started to change my diet; I cut out white sugar, white flour. I would say, at the moment, I'm 95 percent of normal, all through doing things that conventional doctors seem to scoff and laugh at."*[186]

—Robert, who suffered with bipolar disorder for 30 years

With supplementation, she has seen "dramatic improvement in mood," with reduction in depression, irritability, and anxiety; better energy; and amelioration of sleep problems. For most people, tryptophan and 5-HTP have identical effects, she says. "There are a few people who do better on one or the other, but most people do equally well on both." While 5-HTP is available over the counter, tryptophan can only be obtained through a doctor's prescription. As noted previously, however, self-dosing with supplements is not advisable, as everyone is different and it's important to determine exactly what your particular deficiencies and imbalances are.

Tyrosine is sometimes important. "Tyrosine feeds the thyroid as well as the brain," says Ross. As lithium is somewhat suppressive to the thyroid gland, taking tyrosine can provide thyroid support to those people who are on the mood-regulating drug. The people on the severe end of the bipolar disorder spectrum who have come to Ross for treatment are all still on lithium, she reports. They have been able to significantly cut their dosage, however.

"Tyrosine also, at least initially, can increase serotonin," she adds. "But it can be too energizing and stimulating for some who are on the manic end or who cycle rapidly." Ross notes that this can also be true of omega-3 fish oil and flax oil, which can raise dopamine/norepinephrine levels too high.

People with bipolar disorder also need to be careful when it comes to taking glutamine, cautions Ross. Normally, glutamine does not produce an effect on mood, aside from the common report that it makes people "feel even," she says. "That's because it really does burn as fuel, an alternate fuel to glucose. It keeps the blood sugar in the brain really balanced, so you get that even feeling. But it doesn't usually have an emotional tone to it.

"Glutamine can be helpful for people who are in a deep depression," Ross observes. "If they're not, it may not be helpful." With some bipolar people, it eliminates depression and then moves them into mania. Others are not affected in this way. In any case, it is important to be careful with glutamine, she says, noting that her bipolar clients who take it closely monitor their symptoms. "They know themselves, and they don't want to be manic."

Glutamine can be a problem in the case of people who don't know that they have bipolar disorder. "They may come to you for hypoglycemia or diabetes and you give them glutamine, and all of a sudden, you see that they're really buzzing," says Ross. "They may report to you, 'Gee, I feel high on this stuff,' or 'I feel really energetic.' They may not even see it as a negative.

"It's actually a way of inadvertently diagnosing people," Ross notes, because there is "no other condition for which glutamine produces that kind of effect." (The mania brought on by taking glutamine subsides when the person stops taking the supplement.) In cases in which clients have been affected by glutamine in this way, there was no inkling of bipolar disorder in the initial assessment Ross did with them. When she questioned them further, asking if they had ever considered that they might be bipolar, a typical answer was: "I've wondered about that, but I've never been diagnosed with it. I never get that depressed or that manic, but I do have frequent mood swings."

With the proper amino acids, along with a healthful diet with sufficient intake of protein and fat (the good fats such as those found in olive oil and fish), a multivitamin/mineral formula designed to balance blood sugar, an omega-3 fish oil supplement, and other nutrients as indicated, people with bipolar disorder do well, says Ross. As mentioned, eliminating gluten from the diet can also be beneficial, as was true for Darien in the case study to follow.

A Word About Gluten

"The first connection that I made between nutrition and bipolar problems," recalls Ross, "was in the late 1970s when I read several articles about psychiatric hospitals doing experiments removing the gluten-containing grains from the diets of certain randomly selected bipolar patients, and what extraordinary success they had." In her clinic, she has seen enough benefit from this practice in cases of bipolar disorder to recommend that clients try it and see if it makes a difference for them.

123

Gluten is a protein found in wheat, barley, rye, oats, and other cereal grains, and added to many commercial foods. During digestion, this large protein (consisting of long chains of amino acids) is first broken down into smaller peptides before being further reduced into its amino acid components. Peptides are similar to endorphins, substances that athletes know as the source of "runner's high." The peptide form of gluten is called glutemorphin. It is an opioid, meaning that it has an opium-like effect on brain cells.[187]

Gluten is difficult to digest, and many people develop an intolerance to it, which means that the body regards it as a foreign substance and the immune system launches an immune reaction against it. In addition, researchers theorize that incomplete digestion of gluten leads to excessive absorption of glutemorphins from the intestines into the bloodstream, which leads in turn to their passage across the blood-brain barrier where they exert their opioid effects.[188]

In so doing, they depress serotonin, dopamine, and norepinephrine levels in the brain.[189] The opioid aspect also leads people to become addicted to gluten products, notes Ross.

While the intake of carbohydrates in general initially increases serotonin levels, chronic intake dramatically reduces serotonin levels in the brain. Typical results are depression, sleep problems, a craving for carbohydrates, and irritability.[190]

As discussed in chapter 2, allergies can produce mental and behavioral symptoms. This type of allergy or intolerance is termed a brain allergy or a cerebral allergy.

 See Also For more about the role of allergies in bipolar disorder, see chapter 8.

Eating foods that prompt an immune system reaction (foods to which one is sensitive or allergic) can actually interfere with neurotransmitter function. In regard to gluten, research has found that when people who are sensitive to gluten eat food containing it, their neurological function is altered. Depression is one of the manifestations of the alteration, which can occur without people being aware that gluten is a problem for them. Sometimes depression is the only symptom in evidence.[191]

Darien: Amino Acids Stopped the Cycling

Darien, at the age of 40, woke up one morning in the throes of a depression that was so crippling that he couldn't go to work. It was the second week of a new job, for which he had relocated. He loved the new job, but suddenly was unable to do it. Weeks passed and, still not able to work, he lost the job. Before the depression began, he had plans to marry the woman he loved, but the depression brought those plans to a halt as well. "He was just incapacitated," recalls Ross.

Darien had been diagnosed with bipolar disorder and had been cycling between mania and depression for the last 15 years. During the mania, which was severe, he would suddenly jump in his car and drive for thousands of miles, sometimes from one coast to the other, all the way across

Grains that Contain Gluten
wheat
spelt
kamut
teff
triticale
semolina
rye
oats
barley

Foods/Substances that Often Contain Gluten
vinegar
delicatessen meats
bouillon
dextrin
caramel color
food starch
hydrolyzed plant or vegetable protein
monosodium glutamate (MSG)
malt
rice syrup
natural and artificial flavorings

There are many other foods and substances that may contain gluten, including chewing gum, condiments, confectioner's sugar, envelope glue, frozen French fries, ice cream, medications, salad dressings, tomato paste, tuna fish, and vitamin/mineral supplements. Watch for hidden sources of gluten in the diet. Call the manufacturer of a product if you have any doubt.[192]

the country. He would also spend huge sums of money. His mania was also characterized by an extreme personality change. He would be outrageous and loud and pick fights with people—it didn't matter whether they were family, friends, acquaintances, or total strangers. "He just wanted to get into it with people," says Ross. At one point, his behavior in public led to his arrest on charges of disturbing the peace.

Darien took antidepressants at different times and was supposed to be on lithium on a permanent basis, per his doctor's instructions. When he took the lithium, it prevented manic episodes, but he tended to be somewhat depressed all the time and said that on lithium he "just felt flat." Sometimes the depression wasn't as bad as at other times. He finally sought an alternative solution and came to Julia Ross.

Based on his symptom picture, she and her staff nutritionist started him on 5-HTP and glutamine. Later, he took tyrosine on an as-needed basis when he felt his energy was low. As his depression lifted, he stopped taking the glutamine because it began to make him feel manic. Darien also took a multivitamin/mineral supplement and, later, omega-3 essential fatty acids in the form of fish oil. "He felt more focused and more energetic on the omega-3 fatty acids," states Ross. "At one point, however, he took too much fish oil and had a manic reaction that required him to raise his lithium dose briefly." She explains that since he was not depressed, he didn't need as much fish oil and needed to adjust the dosage accordingly.

Within a week of starting this program, Darien's depression began to lift. Within a few months, he could safely say he had moved out of the depressive episode. By the six-month mark, under his physician's supervision, he had cut his lithium dose down to half of what it had been previously.

In Darien's case, it took him a year to go off gluten. He didn't want to give up bread and the other foods that contain gluten, and maintained that it was not a problem for him. Finally, his wife (he had gotten married by then) started pointing out to him that he got diarrhea every time he ate wheat. He had ignored this symptom for years, as many people do. He agreed to try a gluten-free diet for two weeks. Even in that short time, he felt quite a bit better in terms of mood. Nevertheless, he went back on wheat, but the first time he ate it, he had terrible diarrhea.

He got depressed again as well. "The aminos protected him from the depression getting severe, but it was noticeable," says Ross. "He realized it was going to have to be a forever thing. So he began to get really motivated, and he would call manufacturers to find out what was in products because he learned that even a very tiny amount would set him off."

Ross already had him taking a high-potency multivitamin/mineral supplement, along with additional vitamin C. "Whenever somebody has clearly been gluten intolerant, especially with diarrhea, there's a lot of damage to the digestive lining, and they haven't been absorbing nutrients well. We wanted him to get lots of everything." Darien was a good cook and ate three good meals a day, so there was no need for much in the way of dietary changes, aside from eliminating gluten.

It has now been four years since Darien started treatment with Ross. He's still taking the 5-HTP, although much less than at the beginning. "He finds that he needs that still, and feels that he always will," says Ross. "Most people get off the aminos because they no longer need them. They don't even like them after a certain period of time," which is the body's way of telling them that it no longer has a deficiency of amino acids. This pattern applies to most of the people who come to Ross for treatment, "whether they're addicts or suffering from mood-related problems." But someone like Darien, with a severe bipolar problem, is an exception to the rule.

In addition to the 5-HTP, Darien continues to use the other amino acids when he feels he needs them: "a little glutamine if he's feeling like he's sinking into depression," and tyrosine if his energy feels too low. "Since his moods have leveled out, his marriage is much more relaxed and happy," Ross reports. As for his professional life, he started a new career in business and is now working full-time for the first time in 15 years—as a CEO, no less.

7 Restoring the Tempo of Health: Cranial Osteopathy

Structural factors, specifically cranial compression and its far-reaching effects, may also be a component in bipolar disorder. Cranial compression results from distortions in the skull caused by birth trauma or later trauma from injury, emotional stress, vaccinations, medications, or dental factors, such as mercury fillings or root canals, says Linda Garcia, D.D.S., D.M.D., of Schaumberg, Illinois, who specializes in holistic dentistry and cranial osteopathy.

Compression is constriction due to pressure exerted on a body part or system. The impact of cranial compression extends throughout the body, but the immediate effects in the head can be pressure on the brain and cranial nerves, with attendant compromise of neurotransmitter function and brain function in general.

Cranial distortions and compression can be corrected through cranial osteopathy. Dr. Garcia, who frequently works with psychiatric patients, many of whom are referred to her by their psychiatrists, has found that such correction can resolve some cases of bipolar disorder and severe clinical depression, among other conditions.

Dr. Garcia brings a powerful blend of therapeutic traditions to her osteopathic work. Her healing orientation began in her childhood in Brazil, when she discovered that she has what people call "healing hands," the ability to bring about positive changes in an ailment by placing her hands on the person's body. Practicality and family pressure resulted in her directing her healing talents into training in dentistry. She brought a holistic orientation to her work as a dentist, however, and became one of a growing number of dentists who understand the pervasive influence that problems of the teeth and jaw exert on the entire body.

See Also For more about the effects of dental factors, see chapter 3.

Dr. Garcia went on to train in osteopathy. It is not uncommon for dentists to pursue osteopathic training after they learn that problems of the teeth and jaw often arise from distortions in the bones of the skull. She later returned to the energetic healing interest of her childhood and trained with numerous hands-on healers. She also trained with a clairvoyant (a person with psychic abilities) and later studied the Five Levels of Healing and Family Systems Therapy with Dr. Klinghardt (see chapter 2). Her work is now a potent blend of these disciplines.

Cranial Compression from Birth

While cranial distortion can occur through various traumas, a common source is birth trauma resulting from the use of an epidural and the drug Pitocin during childbirth.[193] An epidural block, or epidural for short, is a local anesthetic injected into the space around the lower spinal cord for pain relief during childbirth. Pitocin is the drug given to speed the contractions of labor and hurry the process along. The use of both is common in current obstetrical practice.

While they may be convenient for those involved, these substances can result in the baby's skull being subjected to incredible pressure during birth. Under normal conditions, the woman's pelvis reshapes itself to accommodate birth. This process begins long before the first labor contraction. When the baby drops in late pregnancy, that's already part of the pelvic reshaping. If you anesthetize the pelvis, as with an epidural injection, the reshaping

What Is Cranial Osteopathy?

Osteopathy, or osteopathic medicine, began as a medical discipline in the late 1800s, introduced by physician Andrew Taylor and founded on the principle of treating the whole patient, rather than addressing symptoms on a crisis basis. The interrelationship of anatomy and physiology is central to osteopathy. Manipulation techniques have evolved as hands-on treatment for restoring free movement in the body.[194]

Cranial osteopathy, or osteopathy in the cranial field, was developed by William G. Sutherland, D.O., and is based on an anatomical and physiological understanding of the interrelationship between mechanisms in the skull (cranium) and the entire body.[195] The central component of this relationship is what Dr. Sutherland termed the *primary respiratory mechanism*, or PRM. This is "a palpable movement within the body that occurs in conjunction with the motion of the bones of the head."[196] The flow of cerebrospinal fluid (CSF), the fluid that bathes the brain and spinal cord, is integral to the PRM.

The cranial bones move rhythmically, alternating between expansion and contraction, and this motion is reflected in every cell of the body. Palpable means that the PRM can be felt anywhere in a patient's body by someone who is trained to feel it, that is, a person trained in cranial osteopathy. The PRM can be thought of as the intrinsic fluid drive in the system.

As treatment consists of restoring the full functioning of the PRM in the context of the whole body, it is not restricted to the sacrum, spinal cord, and cranium. Cranial osteopaths use gentle, hands-on manipulation and pressure to release areas of restricted motion. In addition to structural or pain problems, cranial osteopathy can be beneficial for conditions in virtually any system or area of the body, including: behavior problems, seizures, developmental problems, allergies, asthma, frequent colds or sore throats, and irritable bowel syndrome, among many others.[197]

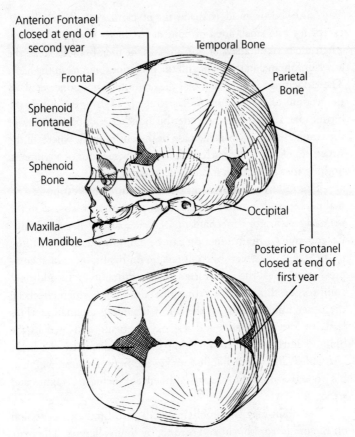

Anterior Fontanel closed at end of second year

Temporal Bone

Frontal

Parietal Bone

Sphenoid Fontanel

Sphenoid Bone

Maxilla

Mandible

Occipital

Posterior Fontanel closed at end of first year

Fontanels of Infant's Skull and the Main Bones of Skull

that normally occurs is inhibited. When labor does not progress because the vital pelvic involvement has been turned off, Pitocin is introduced to force the uterus to contract artificially.

Osteopathic physician Lawrence Lavine, D.O., whose medical roots are in neurology and cranial osteopathy, among other disciplines, describes what follows as "using the child's head as a battering ram to force the pelvis to reshape to accommodate it. . . . Normally in labor, the head comes through, compresses, twists, then extends, and everything opens up. . . . When Pitocin and/or an epidural are used, distortions tend to be locked in."[198]

A newborn's head is made up of cartilage and membrane, except for two small areas of bone at the lower back of the head. There are two fontanels, or openings, in the membranous areas: the anterior fontanel in the front and the posterior fontanel in the back. These openings and the fact that the cranium is not bone yet allow the sections of the skull to overlap so the head can get through the birth canal. Closed fontanels after birth indicate a misalignment of the cranial base, which is the base of the entire skull, where all the structures of the skull attach. If the cranial base is out of alignment, nothing that attaches to it can be in alignment.[199]

The result is compression on the brain, compression of cranial nerves, and systemic effects resulting from disturbance in the primary respiratory mechanism (see sidebar, "What Is Cranial Osteopathy?"). Brain function can be compromised. In addition to the structural effects of compression on the brain, cranial compression may disturb neurotransmitter function.[200] In addition, compression diminishes cerebrospinal fluid flow, which affects all the other fluid systems of the body, including circulation. This leads to fewer nutrients and less oxygen being delivered to the brain.[201] Further, the compression in the skull makes the brain "irritable," and this irritability makes the brain far more vulnerable to adverse environmental influences, including toxins and stress.

The brain may be doubly irritated: first, by the compression on the brain from birth; and second, by brain allergies. The toxic effect of substances (food molecules) not normally found in the bloodstream (as occurs in leaky gut) and continual allergic reaction can irritate the brain as well. In addition, people can develop allergies to their own neurotransmitters. In this case, the body doesn't recognize its own serotonin, for example, instead regarding it as a foreign substance. The feedback mechanism sends the message that more serotonin is needed, so the body just keeps producing it, but the brain is unable to utilize it, which further compromises neurotransmitter function.[202]

 For more about allergies, see chapters 2 and 8.

Fortunately, cranial osteopathy releases the locked state of the skull, restoring it to its natural fluidity, thereby restoring the proper flow of cerebrospinal fluid and the function of the primary respiratory mechanism, removing structurally based interference in neurotransmitter and brain function, and returning balance to the body as a whole.

A case from Dr. Garcia's patient files illustrates how cranial osteopathy and the other therapies she uses came together to reverse long-standing bipolar disorder.

Thomas: No Need to Take Out the Mercury

Thomas, 34 years old, was referred to Dr. Garcia by his psychiatrist to have his mercury dental fillings replaced with non-mercury fillings. The psychiatrist knew of the neurotoxic effect of mercury and felt that it might be contributing to the bipolar disorder from which Thomas had been suffering all his adult life. Muscle testing (see chapters 3 and 8) and hair analysis had revealed high mercury levels.

Until he went on lithium, Thomas had cycled frequently, experiencing deep troughs and severe mania. When he came to Dr. Garcia he had been on both lithium and one antidepressant or another for the past seven years, since getting the diagnosis of bipolar disorder after struggling through most of his twenties not knowing what was the matter with him. Prozac was the latest antidepressant drug he was on.

"The medications were keeping things under control but he was unhappy," recalls Dr. Garcia. He no longer had the mood swings, but he lived in a state of chronic low-grade depression, despite the drugs, psychotherapy, and acupuncture.

While Dr. Garcia has seen dramatic effects on "mental" and other conditions with the removal of mercury or root canals, in many cases she finds that these procedures have to be done after cranial osteopathic treatment in order to produce results. She begins by treating patients osteopathically, in her own approach to healing, and their condition often shifts. That was the case with Thomas, whose mercury removal was then postponed.

133

"As soon as I started treating him, I saw a total shift," she said. What she observed was a change in what she calls his "dissociation." In terms of Dr. Klinghardt's levels of healing, his Physical Body was disconnected or dissociated from his Electromagnetic (Energy) Body. The result was the sense that "he was not present." Dr. Garcia notes that this disconnection is a factor in many of the psychiatric patients she sees.

"Their life force, their potency, their ignition system, as we call it, is depleted," she explains. "It's not being able to recharge itself. Every step of the way, everything is overwhelming. It takes too much out of the body to keep reigniting the system. The life force is not flowing. The body and the person are not working as a whole, but as separate parts. The physical, functional, energetic, and spiritual are disconnected, and of course the medication over time doesn't help much at all. It just gets them addicted and they depend on the medication to overcome their emotional challenges."

Part of their overwhelmed state stems from the fact that their Energy bodies are picking up so much information, according to Dr. Garcia. With the Energy Body dissociated from the Physical Body, they have no boundaries and cannot differentiate the sources of information and what to do with it.

"There are very different degrees of dissociation," she continues. "Some of us have a low degree where we can, by ourselves, without chemicals, come back. At the high degrees, you have schizophrenia." Healing involves reconnecting the Physical, Energy, and Spiritual bodies.

In Thomas' case, osteopathic evaluation revealed that his cerebrospinal fluid (CSF) was not flowing well. "It was almost like his system was stuck. It was slow and pretty toxic." The CSF has its own electromagnetic charge, and when it is not flowing well, that charge is disturbed. This affects the Electromagnetic Body, the potency, throwing it into a state of disorganization. "If that is disorganized, it's the same as if your liver was extremely toxic, your kidneys were not eliminating properly, and your digestive system was totally overwhelmed."

Dr. Garcia's osteopathic focus with Thomas was to reorganize his potency. "When he was in a manic stage, his potency was up, but it was an unbalanced potency. If he were balanced, his potency would not be too high or too low. It would be an average that the system could sustain." Bringing his potency, his Electromagnetic Body, back into an organized state would reconnect it to his Physical Body.

For the first month, Dr. Garcia treated Thomas once a week, and thereafter once every three weeks. Her sessions last between half an hour and an hour and 45 minutes, depending on the information she gets from the body and spirit of each person about what that individual needs at a particular time. Thomas was more present, less dissociated after just one session. His depression began to lift in the weeks that followed, and he wanted to go off his medications.

In her view, his system at that point was strong enough to handle going off the medication, but Dr. Garcia does not advise her patients about the prescription drugs they are taking, as she is neither a physician nor a psychiatrist. Both the psychiatrist and acupuncturist strongly advised Thomas against going off his medications. Given how discontinuation of lithium often catapults people with bipolar disorder into a manic episode, their concern was understandable. Thomas was firm in his resolve, however, and asked Dr. Garcia if his psychiatrist could call her to get a summary of his condition from an osteopathic viewpoint.

They talked, after which the psychiatrist still advised Thomas not to go off his medications, but consented to supervising a gradual decrease in his dosages when he remained adamant. In two months, he had completely stopped taking the drugs. Dr. Garcia continued to treat him and he had no recurrence of either mania or depression. It has now been two years since he began treatment and he is maintaining his stable state, "doing better than ever," reports Dr. Garcia. He also improved his diet during that time and lost 40 pounds, the weight he had gained as a side effect of the lithium.

Family Systems Therapy

Another aspect of Thomas' treatment was to address certain issues through Family Systems Therapy. Dr. Garcia uses Dr.

Klinghardt's method for this, in which it is only necessary to have the patient and practitioner working together to release the transgenerational energetic issues involved in a person's condition. In Thomas' case, Dr. Garcia felt very clearly that there was some foreign female energy occupying his energy field. The presence of this foreign energy was contributing to his dissociation.

The energy was also "dictating a lot in his life, because he was just so open. He didn't have boundaries. You could say that the female energy was using him." You can identify the presence of foreign energies in thoughts and feelings, she notes. "You might be sitting there, and all of a sudden have a thought that comes out of the blue to you. You've got to start to learn if it's your thought or someone else's thought. Or it could be a feeling. You walk into a place and all of a sudden you have a funny feeling, something that doesn't feel right to you." That could be someone else's energy occupying you.

When we take on this energy, Dr. Garcia calls it "carrying other people's bags." By that she means "carrying someone's desires or thoughts or pain." The people whose bags you are carrying could be from a previous generation, which is the basis of Family Systems Therapy. "We carry stuff that's not ours all the time. We don't have the boundaries and the education and the awareness to say, 'Listen, I can only carry one of your bags. I cannot carry four of your bags.' So emotionally, we get overwhelmed, and overcharged by all we are exposed to. We have ten TVs being turned on around us, and we've got to learn how to choose to leave maybe only one channel open instead of ten channels open."

To dispel Thomas' dissociation completely, the female energy needed to be addressed. In his case, identifying the source of that energy was not necessary. It turned out to be enough for Thomas to become aware of it and begin to distinguish between what was his and what was not his, and what bags it was all right with him to continue to carry. The energy was not destructive in itself, but only as it disconnected Thomas from who he really was. Some of the bags he was carrying of this feminine energy fit him well, while others did not. His healing came in discerning the difference. "If he chose to carry someone's bag, it would be his choice, not someone else's choice. In his case, he might have been carrying a little bit more than he could afford to carry," notes Dr. Garcia.

Through becoming aware, Thomas began to make his own choices. With awareness comes reconnection and learning how to be present. Dr. Garcia makes it clear that this process does not involve judging the energy. "There are just different energies around, and you have to be aware of them. At least you have to be aware of why you're feeling the way you are." Learning how to be really present and deciding what you are willing to carry is the key to not being controlled by energies that are not your own.

When someone is in a state of dissociation, those who work with that person on an energetic level have to be responsible about how they do it, Dr. Garcia cautions, both for their own safety and that of the patient. Otherwise, they may take in some of the energies themselves or introduce more foreign energies and cause the person to dissociate even more. "It's the same as going into someone's mouth or blood without wearing gloves and a mask," she explains. Without such protection, AIDS, herpes, or other infections can pass between patient and practitioner.

"The energetic pollution is far worse because we are not educated at all for that," she notes. "People need to be very well trained to do energy work. You've got to be very careful as a practitioner. It's a lot more serious than it looks."

Listening and Healing

Dr. Garcia's first step with patients is to talk with them about what's going on for them. What they say gives her information on both the Physical Level and the Electromagnetic (or energetic, spiritual) Level. Information about the Electromagnetic Level is not so much communicated to her through their words, but in what she picks up telepathically. She then does a hands-on osteopathic evaluation of the person's system, diagnosing how the cerebrospinal fluid is flowing, whether the potency in the system is strong or weak.

She describes her role in treatment as "listening to the information" that the body and spirit of the patient communicate if the practitioner is very still. "You don't dictate anything. You're not going in there and cracking bones and doing all of that," she explains. This is termed being an "efferent practitioner," which is a practitioner who waits for the information to come to her rather than deciding where to work on a patient. It is the body and spirit that dictate the direction that treatment should take, and it is the gift of the doctor to allow this, she says.

Dr. Garcia's particular blend of healing disciplines and abilities makes what she does different from what most other osteopaths do. They have similar training, but her orientation is more to the electromagnetic, spiritual level of osteopathy, while theirs is to the physical level.

For example, in comparing her work with that of a close colleague, a physician who is also an osteopath, she notes that when they check a patient for diagnostic purposes, her tendency is to tap into the potency—the electromagnetic and the spiritual—while his tendency is to tap into the physical first. "He will go to the musculoskeletal and describe that well, whereas I will describe the electromagnetic and the spiritual in more detail," she says. That's not to say that working on the physical level only is not healing, but Dr. Garcia seeks information from both body and spirit for the direction healing should take.

The information arrives silently and comes mostly from what osteopathy calls "the embryo." Osteopathic training involves extensive study in embryology, says Garcia, with the fundamental teaching that "in the first six to eight weeks of embryonic life, there's no genetic or environmental influences at all. The embryo has its own intelligence and is developing on its own."

After that point, genetics and environmental factors begin to influence the developing fetus. Those factors comprise the first "lesion," as it is known in osteopathy, meaning "the first challenge that the embryo has to overcome." According to this model, if the mother is having a difficult time with her spouse, that emotional frequency will only influence the embryo after the first six to eight weeks, and not before.

The initial period in the life of the being, "when the embryo dictates the embryological development, when there is no other influence but its own intelligence and knowing," is the source of the body's wisdom. That is where the information comes from that the practitioner receives regarding how to restore the health of the system. It is "the pure intelligence of the body," which is later obscured and blurred by the toxins of external influences. Dr. Garcia regards this pure intelligence as part of the spirit.

Restoring health is like resetting the timing belt back to its original setting, that is, restoring the system's tempo to what it was in the embryonic stage before genetic and environmental influences intervened. "That tempo is health," says Dr. Garcia.

"I don't ever only treat the symptom," she notes. "I take the patient's whole body to neutral and go from there." Returning to neutral is the first step in restoring the system's natural, original tempo. Being in neutral means that the autonomic nervous system (ANS) is balanced, with neither the parasympathetic nor the sympathetic branch dominant. (The ANS controls the automatic processes of the body such as respiration, heart rate, digestion, and response to stress, with the sympathetic branch being the one involved in the high-adrenaline, fight-or-flight response to stress.)

With the ANS balanced, "the patient gets very calm and the whole system gets very quiet. Then when it's quiet, you've got to be very still as a practitioner, and wait for the health to dictate whatever else needs to be done in this system. It knows exactly what to do in different situations in the body. You're trying to balance the body by bringing that original self-healing ability back into focus. It's gotten so blurry."

It is necessary to synchronize the health at different layers. Therefore, much of osteopathic work entails a purely musculoskeletal orientation, Dr. Garcia says. "Working on the body, you are unlocking the tightness, the rigidity, the obstacles that are keeping the cerebrospinal fluid from being able to flow optimally. Being a dentist, I really focus on the head; that's the cranial osteopathy. I check different parts of the body, but that's where I treat from."

In addition to birth trauma, any other trauma can lock up the system, according to Dr. Garcia. Any physical trauma, such as an accident or fall, emotional trauma, or spiritual trauma shocks the system. The spirit, for example, "may have been so tremendously abused that it's almost having its own life away from the physical." This is the dissociation referred to earlier in the case of Thomas. Spiritual trauma produces the same results as the physical trauma of a serious car accident.

"**Every bone, everything in your system, has to breathe, has to expand and contract to a certain extent. When bones are locked into one position, the system is not breathing enough. By moving the bones, by letting them breathe, everything else breathes, too, from the fluids to the emotions and spirit.**"

Shock to the system causes it to lock up. It can stay that way for a whole lifetime, she notes. In the locked state, the system doesn't breathe or expand. "Every bone, everything in your system, has to breathe, has to expand and contract to a certain extent. When bones are locked into one position, the system is not breathing enough. By moving the bones, by letting them breathe, everything else breathes, too, from the fluids to the emotions and spirit," Dr. Garcia explains.

Many people regard bone as hard, unshapeable, and immovable. On a practical level, this view is belied by what results from osteopathic treatment. Some of Dr. Garcia's patients have come to her for relief from the pain of temporomandibular joint (TMJ) syndrome, which involves misalignment of the teeth and jaw and can produce everything from headaches and neck or back pain to insomnia and depression. TMJ problems are an indication that the bones of the skull are out of alignment, she says. Restoring the skull bones to their proper flexible position may produce noticeable structural changes or not, but a number of TMJ patients say to her after treatment that their teeth come together in a different way than they did before—proof of bone movement.

When you consider the environment in which bones exist in the body, it is a vital milieu. The bones of the head and spine are bathed in cerebrospinal fluid. "Everything is surrounded by life, by liquid, by life force, by the electromagnetic," observes Dr. Garcia. "It's not a stagnant system at all." Regarding the body as purely musculoskeletal is "a very Newtonian perception and understanding of the system, of the body. When you go to Einstein and other wonderful scientists, you start seeing medicine in a totally different way. For example, in quantum physics, if you go down to your very small quantum, it's pure energy. It's an illusion that there's actually any physical to it. So medicine is the same. Some people, a lot of people, are still in the Newtonian knowledge and understanding of the mechanical existence."

The osteopathy that Dr. Garcia practices is a biodynamic model of osteopathy, in which the practitioner doesn't treat just the bone, but the fluids and the potency in the bone, which unlocks everything from the physical to the spiritual. "Once you go deeper into treatments, the structure is just part of it," she says. Restoring the body to its innate tempo, the state of balance and health that existed before genetics and environment intervened, allows the body, mind, and spirit to heal itself. Given the genetic and environmental nature of bipolar disorder, restoring the tempo of health in those who suffer from it can have far-reaching effects.

8 Bipolar Disorder
and Allergies: NAET

"Our psychiatric hospitals might be empty if the causes of our energy blockages could be found and removed," states allergy authority Devi S. Nambudripad, M.D., D.C., L.Ac., Ph.D., of Buena Park, California.[203] Allergic reaction is a primary cause of impeded flow of energy through the body, says Dr. Nambudripad. Often, people are not even aware that they are allergic to something. The allergy goes undetected and the chronic reaction, with its attendant energy blockage, can create a panoply of symptoms, including those of bipolar disorder, clinical depression, and schizophrenia.

Dr. Nambudripad's work has transformed the field of allergy treatment. In the early 1980s, she developed a highly effective, noninvasive, painless method of both identifying and eliminating allergies—NAET (Nambudripad's Allergy Elimination Techniques)—which is now practiced worldwide by more than 5,000 health-care practitioners. Dr. Nambudripad and other NAET practitioners have found that the elimination of allergies can in some cases reverse bipolar disorder and other "mental" illnesses.

Allergy elimination can be beneficial for bipolar disorder in several ways: (1) directly, by removing the source of allergy-related bipolar symptoms; and (2) indirectly, by easing other problems that may be exacerbating or producing symptoms. In the latter category, eliminating allergic reaction improves digestion, which can help reverse the nutrient assimilation and absorption prob-

Symptoms of Allergies

The following are some of the many symptoms and conditions associated with allergies.[204] You can see that they range far beyond the runny nose and teary eyes most often thought of in connection to allergies.

anxiety
attention deficit
Candida/yeast overgrowth
chronic fatigue
craving for carbohydrates/
    chocolate
distractibility
eczema
frequent colds, bronchial infec-
    tions, and other infections
headaches
hyperactivity
hypoglycemia
impulsivity
indigestion

insomnia
irritable bowel syndrome
leaky gut syndrome
mood swings
nervous stomach
obsessive-compulsive disorder
phobias
poor appetite
poor memory
restless leg syndrome
sinusitis
toxicity (reactivity/sensitivity) to
    mercury and other heavy
    metals

lems that may underlie the deficiencies in amino acids, B vitamins, minerals, essential fatty acids, and other nutrients frequently associated with bipolar disorder.

Increased absorption of all nutrients will improve the health of all body systems. Getting rid of allergic reaction also reduces toxic substances in the body, which lifts a burden from the liver and other parts of the detoxification system, leading to more optimal processing of toxins in the future. Finally, allergy elimination lifts a large burden from the immune system, which leads to better overall health.

About NAET

NAET uses kinesiology's muscle response testing (MRT) to identify allergies. Chiropractic and acupuncture techniques are then implemented to remove the energy blockages in the body that underlie allergies, and to reprogram the brain and nervous system not to respond allergically to previously problem substances.

Like many revolutionary inventions, NAET began with an accidental discovery. Dr. Nambudripad, who had long been allergic to nearly everything, one day ate some carrot while she was cooking the two foods she could safely eat—white rice and broccoli. Within moments of eating the carrot, she "felt like [she] was going to pass out."[205] She used muscle response testing to check for an allergy to carrots and was not surprised that she tested highly allergic.

A student of acupuncture at the time, she gave herself an acupuncture treatment, with the help of her husband, to keep from going into shock. She fell asleep with the needles still inserted in specific acupuncture points, and when she woke almost an hour later, she no longer felt sick and tired. In her hand were pieces of the carrot she had been eating. When she repeated the MRT, she no longer tested allergic to carrots. To check the validity of this result, she ate some carrot—no reaction.[206]

Dr. Nambudripad then ate bits of other foods to which she knew she was allergic and her reactions were as they had been— she was still allergic. "[S]o I knew my assumption was correct. My allergy to carrot was gone because of my contact with the carrot while undergoing acupuncture. My energy and the carrot's energy were repelling prior to the acupuncture treatment. After the treatment, their energies became similar—no more repulsion!"[207] She then tried this technique, which she later named NAET, on other foods to which she was allergic. The same thing happened—the allergies disappeared. After many years of living with pervasive allergies, she was able to systematically eliminate them and restore her health.

How NAET Works

NAET is based on the medical model of acupuncture, in which disease is diagnosed and treated as an energy imbalance in one or more of the body's meridians, or energy pathways. These meridians—there are 12 major ones—carry the body's vital energy, or *qi (chi)*, to organs and throughout the system. Acupuncturists rebalance a meridian's energy by treating acupoints, the points on the body's surface that correspond to that meridian. Via the painless insertion of needles or the application of pressure, the acupuncturist can remove energy blockages, get stagnant energy moving, or calm an overactive energy meridian.

According to Dr. Nambudripad, who is a licensed acupuncturist, allergies are "energy incompatibilities" that create energy blockages in the body. That is, the body's energy field regards the energy field of a substance—eaten, inhaled, or otherwise contacted—as incompatible with its own, and its presence disturbs the flow of energy along the body's meridians. One, several, or even all of the meridians may be affected. The central nervous system records the energy disturbance and is then programmed to regard the substance as toxic. NAET uses chiropractic and acupuncture techniques to restore the smooth flow of energy along the meridians and reprogram the central nervous system to no longer regard the substance as incompatible energetically.

Muscle Response Testing

The energy disturbance created by an allergy is the key to muscle response testing. To be tested for a potential allergen (something that causes an allergic reaction), you hold a vial containing the substance in one hand. You hold your other arm straight out in front of you, and attempt to keep it there while the person testing pushes down on it slightly. Normally, you can easily hold your arm in place, but when you are allergic to the substance in the vial, your muscle response is weakened by the energy disturbance the allergy causes. A weakened response in testing indicates a possible allergy.

Those who have not experienced this test often find it difficult to believe that it can tell you anything, much less identify allergies. Upon undergoing the test, however, most people are amazed to discover that their arm seems to have a life, or mind, of its own. One moment, while holding one test substance, they see their arm drop slightly, and the next, with a different test vial,

In Their Own Words

"Our daughter was diagnosed with bipolar disease in 1981. She became ill while in her first year of college out-of-state, and at the end of the year we took her home in a suicidal depression. After seeing psychologists and getting no help, we finally had to have her hospitalized, as she seemed intent on killing herself. In the state hospital, she was diagnosed with manic depression with schizoaffective disorder. She was in the hospital for four months, came home heavily drugged, and was again hospitalized seven months later for another three months."

After that, she was "hospitalized every 10 or 11 months for anywhere from 7 to 11 weeks at a time. . . . After a couple of years on this merry-go-round, we began to look into alternative therapies. . . . "

When her acupuncturist suggested NAET, "my response was 'but she is not allergic to anything.' You see, she had never exhibited any of the usual signs of allergic reaction." When the acupuncturist said that she was a highly allergic person, "I didn't really believe her, but we decided to give it a try, since we felt that we had nothing to lose. So

the arm holds steady. The person being tested usually does not know what's in the vial, so that does not influence the outcome.

For the treatment phase, the person holds the vial of the offending substance while the NAET practitioner uses slight pressure, needles, or a chiropractic tool to treat the appropriate points to clear the affected meridian(s). Keeping the vial in your energy field during this process reprograms the brain and nervous system to regard the substance as innocuous. In general, it is then necessary to avoid ingesting or otherwise having contact with the substance for 25 hours after treatment.

Dr. Nambudripad explains the reason for this time period: "An energy molecule takes 24 hours to travel through the body completing its circulation through all 12 major meridians, their branches, and sub-branches. It takes two hours to travel through one meridian. . . . When the allergy is treated through NAET, the patient has to wait 24 hours to let the energy molecule carrying *she began NAET treatments. She has, through the past 16 years, been on numerous antipsychotic, antimanic, and anticonvulsive medications, and on extremely high doses each time she was hospitalized, as her manic and schizoid episodes were so profound. Now, 18 months after beginning the NAET treatments, our daughter is off all but a very small amount of her last remaining medication. . . .*

"At the present time our daughter is working at a local library, and once more is reading two or three books at a time. Until now, she has been unable to read more than a few lines at a given time, because her mind was so cloudy from a combination of drugs and the illness. . . .

"Our daughter is 36 years old, and it's as if her life is just beginning. The prognosis is that she will be off all medication within the next three to four months. We are lowering her medications very slowly, in spite of the fact that she has exhibited barely any symptoms of withdrawal, thanks to the alternative methods, in addition to the NAET, that are being employed."[208]

—Helene and Fred, parents of a recovered daughter

the new information pass through the complete cycle of the journey."[209]

To be safe, one hour is added to the 24-hour cycle. If the person eats the allergenic food or has contact with an allergenic substance before the cycle is complete, the clearing treatment will likely have to be repeated and the food or other substance will need to be avoided for another 25 hours.

Common Allergens

You can have sensitivities or allergies to anything you eat, drink, inhale, or touch or are touched by, such as fabric, cosmetics, chemicals, and environmental pollutants. Many people are allergic to the same basic substances. In many cases, people are not aware of their allergies. They may even crave the food or other substance that they are allergic to.

"An allergy can manifest as an addiction or an aversion," explains Dr. Nambudripad. "It can go either way. I treat people with addictions for allergies because they're allergic to something that is causing them to be addicted to the substance." Once you clear that allergy, the addiction disappears, she says. Conversely, some people strongly dislike certain foods or other items and they are actually allergic to them. After you clear the allergy, the aversion is gone as well.

For the purposes of clearing people of their allergies more quickly, NAET combines the most common allergens in five basic groups: egg mix (egg white, egg yolk, chicken, and the antibiotic tetracycline); calcium mix (breast milk, cow's milk, goat's milk, milk albumin, casein, lactic acid, calcium, and coumarin, a phenolic or natural component found in milk); vitamin C (fruits, vegetables, vinegar, citrus, and berry); B complex vitamins (17 vitamins in the B family); and sugar mix (cane, corn, maple, grape, rice, brown, and beet sugars, plus molasses, honey, fructose, dextrose, glucose, and maltose).

You may wonder why tetracycline is included in the egg mix. The answer is that chickens are routinely fed this antibiotic to keep infections that might kill them from doing so and also to prevent the spread of infection from chicken to chicken. Thus, tetracycline is a component of commercial chicken products and, as such, it has become a common allergen.

For some people, it is sufficient to clear the five basic groups, but most people with severe conditions such as bipolar disorder have more extensive allergies. The larger basic collection of allergens includes magnesium, essential fatty acid oils, amino acids, grain mix (including gluten), yeast mix (including acidophilus), artificial sweeteners, food additives, and food coloring, among others. A number of these substances have implications for bipolar disorder.

Deficiencies in magnesium, essential fatty acids, and amino acids are common among people with bipolar disorder. If a person is allergic to a nutrient, the body cannot absorb it and thus becomes deficient in it. An allergy to these nutrients might explain the deficiencies. An allergy to gluten (a grain protein) could also contribute to the amino acid deficiency common in bipolar disorder, as the body cannot properly digest this food and therefore cannot assimilate the amino acids it contains.

As noted in chapter 2, digestive problems have an impact on the brain. An allergy to acidophilus means that this beneficial bacteria is unable to perform its function of keeping the *Candida* population in the intestines in check. The result is digestive dysfunction.

Artificial sweeteners, food additives, and food coloring contain chemicals that are neurotoxic to some individuals. NAET practitioners would say that the neurotoxicity stems from the fact that the individuals are allergic to the substances. Once cleared of the allergy, in most cases, people can eat foods containing these additives without suffering the negative effects. The same is true of gluten and casein (in the calcium mix), which is good news for those who have struggled with a gluten-free and/or casein-free diet.

It is worthwhile to note at this point that people can develop allergies to anything, even to nutrients that are natural to and required by the body. Says Dr. Nambudripad, "Any substance under the sun, including sunlight itself, can cause an allergic reaction in any individual."[210] The body can even develop a reactivity to its own tissue and brain chemicals, such as an allergy to one's own brain, hypothalamus, nerves, lung tissue, and neurotransmitters such as serotonin.

 For more about allergies to neurotransmitters, see chapter 7.

The Nature of Allergies

Allergic reactions tend to affect certain organs or meridians in individuals, depending on where their weak or vulnerable areas are, says Dr. Nambudripad. The organ most affected is known as the "target organ." The weakness can be genetic in nature or created by environmental factors such as toxic exposure or lack of adequate nutrition. The target organ can be the nervous system or the brain. If that is the case, chronic allergic reaction can negatively affect brain and nervous system function.

In the case of food allergies, "with the first bite of an allergic food, the brain begins to block the energy channels, attempting to prevent the adverse energy of the food from entering into the body," says Dr. Nambudripad.[211] Chronic blockage of the Stomach meridian can also affect brain function. Manic disorders, depressive disorders, and schizophrenia are among the manifestations of this blockage. When the liver is the target organ or the Liver meridian is blocked, emotional imbalances, anger, mood swings, and depression are among the outcomes.[212]

As for how the allergies or sensitivities develop in the first place, Dr. Nambudripad cites heredity, toxins, weakened immunity, emotional stress, overexposure to a substance, and radiation. Anything that causes energy blockages in the body, which throws off the body's electromagnetic field, can cause an allergy to develop, she says. Toxins of any kind, from the neurotoxin mercury to the by-products of bacterial infection, disturb energy flow, as do synthetic food additives and artificial sweeteners.

The electromagnetic fields (EMFs) of televisions, computers, and other electrical devices in the house are a common culprit in the development of allergies, according to Dr. Nambudripad. The practice of feeding infants and children in front of the television so they will keep quiet and cooperate can be a recipe for allergies. The television's EMF extends at least 20 feet, she notes, and throws off the child's own energy field. You could say that it "short-circuits the energy patterns," she says. And it does so while the child is eating, which is akin to doing NAET in reverse, programming the child to be allergic to that food.

NAET removes the energy blockages underlying allergies, which returns the individual's electromagnetic field to its normal state. In the following two cases, NAET reversed severe bipolar disorder by eliminating the many allergies from which the people suffered, unbeknownst to them.

Delia: 170 Allergies

Delia, now 46, had a major breakdown at the age of 16, received the dual diagnosis of manic-depressive disorder and schizophrenia, and was hospitalized. She was in the hospital for 17 years, and treated with shock therapy and drugs.

At the age of 32, she was released from the hospital. She was on lithium and other psychiatric medications. The lithium kept her violent and angry episodes only somewhat under control. She still experienced periods when she would explode in anger. Her family was having a very difficult time with her.

Delia's mother had come to Dr. Nambudripad for pain and skin problems, both of which had been resolved by NAET. She asked her to treat Delia. Dr. Nambudripad wasn't sure that she could help her, not because she didn't think NAET would improve her condition, but because Delia, with her anger and violent tendencies, was such an extreme case to handle in a clinic situation. If she were treating Delia in a hospital, Dr. Nambudripad would not have hesitated. But Delia's mother wanted desperately to try it, so they did.

In the beginning, when Delia came into Dr. Nambudripad's clinic for her NAET treatments, she would fight with all the office staff, and everyone was scared of her. One or both of her parents always accompanied her, until later in her treatment when she no longer had violent outbursts and was able to come in on her own.

From the very beginning, Delia submitted to NAET without protest or resistance. "For some reason, she took a liking to me," recalls Dr. Nambudripad. "We got along fine. The rest of the office staff was afraid, but I wasn't afraid. She knew that something was going to happen here, so she stuck with me, and became one of our best patients."

Delia needed many, many treatments. It took four years to clear her of all of her allergies, and sometimes she was getting treatments three days a week. Dr. Nambudripad notes that hers was a very extreme case; the number of treatments she required was far beyond what is normally needed. She had a host of allergies, most of which took multiple treatments to clear, instead of the usual single treatment. In the case of chemicals, pesticides, insulation, materials in her own house, including the paint, and other environmental allergens, it took many, many treatments to clear each one. She had around 170 allergies in all.

Despite the daunting prospect of clearing all these allergies, she never quit, says Dr. Nambudripad. Within the first two months, she could see that her condition was improving and so she stuck with it. "She was very, very faithful to treatment. Now, if she feels that she has an allergic reaction to something, she immediately comes to our office and gets treated. She knows this is the only thing to help her so far."

At the end of four years of NAET treatment, she was off all of her medications. She was doing yoga exercises twice a day, eating a healthful diet, and taking vitamin and mineral supplements. Dr. Nambudripad encourages people with bipolar disorder "to get involved with yoga, meditation, or such disciplines to help maintain their mental balance. They also should check their vitamin B complex and trace mineral levels periodically and continue to take these nutrients as needed because they can become deficient very quickly."

Delia got a full-time job and wanted to go off the permanent disability everyone thought she would be on for the rest of her life. Dr. Nambudripad suggested that she have the disability put on hold, rather than cancelled, so she could go back on it if she ever needed to. Delia agreed, but in the five years since then, she has still not needed it. Both Delia and her mother consider Delia to be fully recovered.

Bruce: Fast-Food Nightmare

Bruce, 44, also had a dual diagnosis of bipolar disorder and schizophrenia. He had just graduated with high honors from a prestigious university when he became sick. He had been unable to resume his life since then. When he came to Dr. Nambudripad in his early forties, he was on three or four different drugs and in worse shape than Delia had been.

"Sometimes when I treated certain things, his head would feel like it was exploding," Dr. Nambudripad recalls. "He would hit his head on the wall and on the floor." At times during the first two weeks of treatment, he got so violent that she had to give him an injection. His family was highly supportive of NAET, and his mother, a nurse, always accompanied her son.

Bruce got NAET treatments two or three times a week. After the first two difficult weeks, he was calmer and felt better, and there were no more problems during treatment. In his case, there were around 80 allergies that needed to be cleared, but they cleared more easily than Delia's allergies did. His were mainly food allergies. He was highly allergic to orange juice, sugar, minerals, and all the gluten grains, especially wheat. He was also very allergic to fat. "He used to crave fatty foods, like fried fast foods, with those terrible hydrogenated oils and additives," says Dr. Nambudripad. "He used to go and eat at Carl's Jr., and that day would be the worst nightmare for the family." His allergy would plunge him into an episode.

Bruce had two years of treatment, at the end of which he was back to what he considered to be about 80 percent normal. "He was doing very well; he could drive, he could do a lot of things on his own. He was working in the family business again, as he used to do." Dr. Nambudripad taught Bruce's mother how to do NAET, so if any allergies arose, she could treat him.

Now, three years later, Bruce is "100 percent normal," no longer takes any psychiatric medications, and is highly successful in the business world. Like Delia, he practices yoga regularly, takes vitamins and minerals, and eats healthfully.

9 Rebalancing the Vital Force: Homeopathy

Like acupuncture, homeopathy is an energy medicine. Homeopathic medicines do not contain biochemical components of the plants or other substances from which they are derived, but rather transfer their energetic patterns. The medicines help restore the individual's energy (or vital force, or *qi*) to its natural equilibrium and thus return balance to the body, mind, and spirit. With disturbed energy flow an underlying factor in bipolar disorder, homeopathy can be a highly useful treatment.

Judyth Reichenberg-Ullman, N.D., L.C.S.W., of Edmonds, Washington, is an internationally known naturopathic and homeopathic physician. She went into homeopathy because of her interest in mental health. In her early career as a psychiatric social worker, she worked on a locked psychiatric ward, in emergency rooms, nursing homes, halfway houses, and patients' homes. "I saw the whole spectrum, and the suffering was terrible," she recalls. "I didn't see conventional medicine as having a magic bullet for most of these people. With the degree of side effects they were experiencing [from medications], I thought there must be something better."[213]

Dr. Reichenberg-Ullman discovered that "something better" in homeopathy, as did her husband, Robert Ullman, N.D. They now teach, lecture, and have written numerous books together, including *Prozac Free: Homeopathic Alternatives to Conventional*

154

Drug Therapies. Their column on homeopathic treatment has run in the esteemed journal *Townsend Letter for Doctors and Patients* since 1990.

They wrote *Prozac Free* to share their discovery of an effective alternative to medications for depression, bipolar disorder, and other psychiatric disorders. "As shown by the numerous patients we have treated successfully, we believe we have found a method that can transform the lives of many people," she states.[214] "Certainly homeopathy can't help everybody, but the number of people that can be helped with these impairing mental and emotional conditions is incredibly gratifying."

Another homeopath, who is also a psychiatrist, has this to say about homeopathy's effectiveness in his foreword to *Prozac Free*: "In my 30 years as a psychiatrist I have found over and over again that nothing can match homeopathy in efficacy for treating mental and emotional illness when the provider of homeopathic treatment is a well-trained and competent classical homeopath," states Michael R. Glass, M.D., of Ithaca, New York. "Even in those cases where we cannot take the patient off psychiatric drugs, we usually can reduce the dosage and thereby decrease uncomfortable side effects, while at the same time producing real improvements in functioning."[215]

Not only is homeopathy effective, but it is also safe and long-lasting, says Dr. Reichenberg-Ullman. It has the further potential benefit of alleviating physical problems along with the mental/emotional symptoms[216] for which someone with bipolar disorder seeks treatment. This is because homeopathy addresses the underlying imbalance that is responsible for all of a person's symptoms. The imbalance occurs on an energetic level, which is why an energy medicine such as homeopathy is so effective in restoring balance. Let's look more closely at the concept of energy imbalance.

Bipolar Disorder and the Vital Force

We are energetic organisms, or energy-modulated organisms, explains Dr. Reichenberg-Ullman, and that energy is our vital force or *qi*, as it is known in traditional Chinese medicine. "The vital force of each person, because of their makeup, has a certain susceptibility. Due to that susceptibility there are going to be certain factors that trigger an imbalance or symptoms in that person."

For example, in a family in which one parent has bipolar disorder, which research has shown to have a genetic component, one of the children develops the illness and the others don't. That one child was susceptible in some way. The same is true of nonpsychiatric illnesses, Dr. Reichenberg-Ullman points out, citing epidemics as an example. Even in virulent epidemics, there are people who are not susceptible and do not contract the illness, she notes.

Even with a susceptibility, or vulnerability, a triggering factor may not necessarily tip the balance into a manic or depressive episode unless the person's vital force is compromised. "It's important to realize that the vital force or the energetic equilibrium of that individual is the bottom line," says Dr. Reichenberg-Ullman. "When there is an imbalance, a disturbance underneath the surface of the lake, then there are ripples that go out. Those ripples can manifest in any number of ways. One of those ripples could end up being a biochemical imbalance, an imbalance in neurotransmitters."

Scientific consensus currently holds that neurotransmitter problems are the factor behind bipolar disorder, depression, and other mental illnesses. In actuality, the research supporting this is "still more theoretical than they would make it out to be," says Dr. Reichenberg-Ullman. In her view, a deeper imbalance in a person's energetic equilibrium is what throws neurotransmitter supply and function out of balance.

Thus, simply attempting to correct the neurotransmitter problem is not getting to the real source of the mental disorder. "You have to deal with that underlying disturbance, or else it's like putting your finger in the dike, which I think is what, to a large degree, conventional medicine is doing." She cites the use of Prozac as an example of putting the finger in the dike.

Like many natural medicine physicians, Dr. Reichenberg-Ullman regards symptoms, whether mental, emotional, or physical, as an individual's attempt to cope with the underlying disturbance. The body has its own wisdom, and symptoms are the ways in which a particular person adapts to the imbalance in their vital force. The beauty of homeopathy is that it goes to the heart of the matter and corrects the disturbance in the vital force. From that, all the other imbalances, including neurotransmitter and hormonal problems, correct as well. This is why homeopathy can address both your bipolar disorder and whatever physical problems you are manifesting.

> **Dr. Reichenberg-Ullman regards symptoms, whether mental, emotional, or physical, as an individual's attempt to cope with the underlying disturbance. The body has its own wisdom, and symptoms are the ways in which a particular person adapts to the imbalance in their vital force.**

Standard conventional tests have revealed the changes that transpire on the physical level, notes Dr. Reichenberg-Ullman. For example, she has seen cases of an overactive or underactive thyroid, as identified by tests that measure thyroid function, in which a second test taken after classical homeopathic treatment showed that the condition had reversed itself. She has seen similarly beneficial results in the red blood cell counts in people who prior to homeopathic treatment were anemic.

What Is Homeopathy?

To understand *homeopathy*, it is helpful to consider the derivation of the word as well as that of *allopathy*, both of which were coined by the father of homeopathy, Dr. Samuel Hahnemann, in the late 1700s. A German physician and chemist who became increasingly frustrated with conventional medical practice, Dr. Hahnemann devoted himself to developing a safer, more effective approach to medicine. The result was homeopathy, which arose out of his discovery that illness can be treated by giving the patient a dilution of a plant that produces symptoms resembling those of the illness when given to a healthy person.

This principle, "let likes be cured with likes," became known as the Law of Similars. Dr. Hahnemann named this system of healing "homeopathy," a combination of the Greek *homoios* (similar) and *pathos* (suffering). At the same time, he dubbed conventional medicine "allopathy," which means 'opposite suffering,' to reflect that model's approach of treating illness by giving an antidote to the symptoms, a medicine that produces the opposite effect from what the patient is suffering. (A laxative for constipation is an illustration of the allopathic approach; it produces diarrhea.)[217]

Homeopathic remedies can be employed as a simple remedy to address a certain transitory ailment or as a constitutional remedy to address the whole cluster of physical, psychological, and emotional characteristics—the constitution—of an individual patient. A constitutional remedy works to restore balance and thus health on all levels.

Homeopathic remedies are prepared through a process of dilution of plant, mineral, or animal substances, which results in a "potentized" remedy, one that contains the energy imprint of the substance rather than its biochemical components. This is why homeopathy falls into the category of energy medicine; it works on an energetic level to effect change in all aspects of a person and restore balance to the whole.

Paradoxically, the higher the number of dilutions, the greater the potency and the effects of the remedy. Thus the higher the potency number, the more powerful the remedy. Remedies used to treat a transitory condition are usually 6C, 12C, or 30C, relatively low-potency remedies. A constitutional remedy is often a 200C potency, which means it has been diluted 200 times (99 parts alcohol or water to one part substance), or a 1M potency, which means it has been diluted a thousand times.

The Benefits of Homeopathic Treatment

Dr. Reichenberg-Ullman cites the following benefits of constitutional homeopathic treatment.[218] Homeopathy:

- treats the whole person

- treats the root of the problem

- treats each person as an individual

- uses natural, nontoxic medicines

- is considered safe and does not have the side effects of prescription drugs

- heals physical, mental, and emotional symptoms

- uses medicines, one dose of which works for months or years rather than hours

- uses inexpensive medicines

- is cost effective.

Constitutional Treatment of Bipolar Disorder

Classical or constitutional homeopathic treatment is distinct from the use of homeopathic remedies for acute symptoms in that it employs a single remedy that addresses the particular and unique mental, emotional, and physical state of an individual. Dr. Reichenberg-Ullman explains it this way: "Each child, or adult, is much like a jigsaw puzzle. Once all of the pieces are assembled in their proper places, an image emerges that is distinct from other puzzles. It is the task of a homeopath to recognize that image and to match it to the corresponding image of one specific homeopathic medicine."[219]

The homeopath makes that match by considering the person's behaviors, feelings, attitudes, beliefs, likes, dislikes, physical symptoms, prenatal and birth history, family medical history, eating and sleeping patterns, and even dreams and fears.[220] By giving the remedy whose qualities match this unique cluster most closely, the homeopathic principle of "like cures like" is put into operation and the remedy works to restore the person to balance. People may have one constitutional remedy that is their match throughout their life, or it may change over time and a different constitutional remedy might then be required.

Homeopathy does not prescribe according to diagnostic labels, but rather according to the complete picture of the individual. Thus, there is no universal remedy for bipolar disorder, and two people suffering from this condition will likely require two entirely different remedies, chosen from more than two thousand possible homeopathic remedies.

It's interesting to note that the qualities of the remedy that is the correct one for a person reflect his areas of susceptibility or vulnerability.

"When a certain homeopathic medicine benefits a person, that tells me something about that person," observes Dr. Reichenberg-Ullman. "From understanding that homeopathic medicine, I know what kinds of conditions, whether mental, emotional, or physical, that the person is likely to be susceptible to and what kinds they aren't. It often gives you a predictive capacity. Conventional medicine doesn't understand people deeply enough in most cases to be able to do that."

A single dose of a constitutional remedy is sometimes all that is needed at first (though the remedy may also be given more often, even daily). When the remedy is the correct one for an individual, changes can begin relatively quickly, within two to five weeks after taking the dose. (Some people experience changes in the first day, or even within hours.) If there are no changes within five weeks, that generally indicates that it is not the proper remedy. A remedy continues to work over time, anywhere from four months to a year or longer. Repeat doses may be necessary if there is a relapse of symptoms, or sometimes a different remedy may be called for.

Due to the way homeopathic remedies work, it is important to continue treatment for one to two years at least, states Dr. Reichenberg-Ullman. This does not necessarily entail frequent appointments with your homeopath, however. As stated, a single dose of a remedy works for some time; this is also true of a daily remedy.

While certain substances (notably coffee, menthol, camphor, and eucalyptus) can antidote single-dose homeopathic remedies in some sensitive individuals, prescription medications may not interfere with their function. (Topical steroids, antibiotics, and antifungals and oral antibiotics and cortisone products can be suppressive and are best used in consultation with your homeopath.[221]) Be assured, however, that homeopathic remedies do not interfere with the function of conventional medicine. Thus, you can pursue homeopathic treatment while continuing your medications or working with your prescribing doctor to phase them out when possible.

As a final note, regarding the efficacy of homeopathy in treating bipolar disorder, Dr. Reichenberg-Ullman states, "Homeopathic effectiveness is most limited by the skill, knowledge, and experience of the homeopath and the cooperation of the patient. The theory works, but it must be applied well and for a long enough time with sufficient expertise to produce results."[222]

In her experience, less severe mood swings, as in cyclothymia, and hormonally generated mental and emotional states have an excellent response to homeopathy, as does mild to moderate depression. Classical bipolar disorder and obsessive-compulsive disorder are frequently responsive to homeopathy. In the case of bipolar, the person may need to remain on lithium, but may be able to reduce the dosage under the guidance of the prescribing physician.

One particular patient of Dr. Reichenberg-Ullman's is still on lithium, but has had no hospitalizations since she began homeopathic treatment over five years ago. "And she's been through major life stresses," which before treatment would have sent her into the hospital, despite the lithium. Homeopathy has balanced out her system so "she can withstand stresses in her life that many people with bipolar disorder cannot."

The results she has seen with bipolar disorder and other "mental" illnesses have given Dr. Reichenberg-Ullman a vision for the future. She would like to see homeopathy become standard treatment in both inpatient psychiatric facilities and emergency rooms. In the latter, homeopathy could be used "across the whole spectrum, for everything from trauma to acute psychiatric disturbances," she notes.

There are more than one thousand classical homeopaths in the United States, a small percentage of whom specialize in mental health. One source to help you find a qualified homeopath in your area is the Homeopathic Academy of Naturopathic Physicians (HANP), 12132 SE Foster Place, Portland, OR 97266; tel: 503-761-3298; website: www.healthy.net/hanp.

Joyce: On Tiger Lily, Off Depakote and Paxil

When Joyce, 33, came to Dr. Reichenberg-Ullman for treatment, she had been on lithium for ten years.* Her troubles began with anxiety, depression, and insomnia when she was 14, but did not escalate into "mental" illness until her senior year when a "hyper" episode prompted her expulsion from high school. Soon after, she got pregnant and had an abortion, which resulted in her passing large blood clots for a time afterward.

"Then I became really psychotic," Joyce recalls. "I was sent to the psychiatric wards of three different hospitals." The doctors, diagnosing her as schizophrenic, gave her Haldol and a number of other medications. Joyce's condition worsened on the drugs, and the doctors eventually took her off them.

Out of the hospital at last, she struggled with severe depression for months. Later, she managed to complete a course in interior decorating, but four months afterward had another breakdown. This time, she was diagnosed with bipolar disorder and put on lithium, but she managed to stay out of the hospital.

---

*This case study adapted, by permission of Judyth Reichenberg-Ullman, N.D., L.C.S.W., from her book with coauthor Robert Ullman, N.D., *Prozac Free: Homeopathic Alternatives to Conventional Drug Therapies* (Berkeley, CA: North Atlantic Books, 2002), pages 195-9.

Other manic episodes followed, but the one that sent her to homeopathic treatment came when she was 32. She was in art school at the time and having difficulty focusing. She was drinking a lot of coffee, smoking, and going out at night. The episode began after she had finished her last exam and had only one more paper to write. In retrospect, she can see the signs of increasing mania, but she didn't notice it at the time. She stayed up most of the night working on the paper.

From the next day on, Joyce escalated into the worst manic episode she had ever had. It lasted for months. "I destroyed my life," she says. "I blew all of my savings. I bought a boat but had nowhere to put it. I left my job, took all of my things, and drove to Florida for two weeks. I charged it all to my credit card." Then she threw away all her clothes, burned all paper reminders of the past, and flew to the Caribbean. She slept with strangers and went on another buying binge, purchasing expensive clothing and jewelry.

Six months later, she crashed. She declared bankruptcy, lost her car, and had another abortion. She got by on a low-paying job, food stamps, and help from her parents. Barely functioning, Joyce felt "as if she were dying." She had stopped taking her lithium. It wasn't long before she was back in the hospital, but since she didn't have health insurance, she was only there for one night.

When Joyce came to Dr. Reichenberg-Ullman, she characterized her mental state as being "in a fog" and "hanging on by a thread." Her physical symptoms included a feeling of weakness as from loss of muscle tone, chronic psoriasis, lack of menstruation since the abortion six months prior, increased facial and body hair, recurring vaginal infections, leaking after urination, and terrible digestion. Later, she reported that she had also been having night sweats. She had just started on Paxil for depression and Depakote in an attempt to stabilize her moods, but she objected to these drugs because she said they caused hair loss, so she was looking for another solution for her bipolar disorder.

Joyce's constitutional homeopathic remedy was *Lilium tigrinum* (derived from tiger lily). This remedy is indicated "predominately for women with hormonal problems who have a wild feeling inside and frequently a conflict between their spiritual and sexual natures," says Dr. Reichenberg-Ullman.

Joyce's symptoms began to improve within a month. Her moods felt more stable and she was sleeping better. It is not possible to determine whether this improvement was the result of her homeopathic remedy or the psychiatric medications. If the remedy was working, however, it would be expected that her periods would return, notes Dr. Reichenberg-Ullman, which they did in three months from the start of treatment. This meant that the remedy had helped her body restore the hormonal imbalance that her symptoms clearly evidenced.

In her second follow-up appointment, six weeks after the first, Joyce reported that her anxiety and panic had disappeared and her night sweats had nearly stopped. Her psoriasis was under control. Under her psychiatrist's supervision, she had stopped taking the Depakote.

By seven months from the start of homeopathic treatment, Joyce was tapering off the Paxil, again, with her psychiatrist's oversight. She reported that her moods had stabilized; she was "neither depressed nor destitute," she said. She was feeling much better in general, had had four normal periods, and her digestion was improved.

Sandy: Homeopathic Lithium

Sandy, 44, diagnosed with bipolar disorder and borderline depression, had a history of suicide attempts.* The first was when she was 14 years old. It was not long after her boyfriend at the time had broken up with her, and she had gone from "one relationship to another looking for love." One night, after her mother got angry at her for staying out too late, she "took a bottle of antibiotics on impulse," she says.

---

*This case study adapted, by permission of Judyth Reichenberg-Ullman, N.D., L.C.S.W., from her book with coauthor Robert Ullman, N.D., *Prozac Free: Homeopathic Alternatives to Conventional Drug Therapies* (Berkeley, CA: North Atlantic Books, 2002), pages 187-90.

Impulsivity and the "horrible pit" of severe depressions plagued her life from then on and were deeply disturbing to her. In her case, lithium proved unhelpful, and over the years she took "more medications than I can even remember." She cites her impulsiveness as responsible for her being scattered, having trouble sticking with anything, changing jobs frequently, and conducting relationships characterized by turmoil.

"I'm impulsive in my attention, parenting, eating, spending," Sandy told Dr. Reichenberg-Ullman during the initial intake. "You name it and I do it impulsively. . . . I have a shotgun approach to everything." Her impulsivity led to overspending and financial disaster. Angry outbursts were also a characteristic of this end of the mood spectrum.

She experienced drastic fluctuations between the impulsivity and anger, with its debilitating effects in her life, and deep depression, which was debilitating in a different way and made her feel trapped. Her third suicide attempt came after the death of her mother, who was "the pillar of her life." With her mother gone, Sandy felt as though a door had slammed shut and a part of herself had died, too.

Fortunately, Sandy survived the attempt, but it was not until ten years later that she found a solution to her problems in homeopathic treatment. At that point, she was on the antidepressants Zoloft and Paxil, along with Ambien for when she had trouble sleeping. Her mood swings were still running her life.

In getting the complete symptom picture of Sandy, Dr. Reichenberg-Ullman learned that while she liked being a mother (of two children), she resented having to mother her husband. She was afraid of falling and of the dark, and had "vivid, disturbing dreams about ghosts, of fighting evil forces, and of losing her soul." Insomnia was an ongoing problem, as was biting her nails, which she had been doing all her life. Her food cravings ran to very salty French fries and bread with butter. Stimulants such as caffeine and amphetamines held a strong attraction for her.

On a physical level, her libido was very low, she suffered from premenstrual irritability, and had a rash near her lips. Hot weather made her feel nauseous and gave her a headache and diarrhea.

Dr. Reichenberg-Ullman prescribed *Lithium muriaticum* (derived from lithium chloride), as indicated by "her debilitating impulsivity, changeable nature, history of manic and depressive episodes, issues with mothering and her own mother, food cravings, and aggravation from the sun."

It is important to note here that homeopathic *Lithium* is not necessarily indicated for people who have received a bipolar diagnosis. Again, remedies are not prescribed based on diagnostic labels. Bipolar disorder, like any other condition, is highly variable in the homeopathic medicines indicated in individual cases. *Lithium* is actually not a very common remedy, says Dr. Reichenberg-Ullman. It just happened that Sandy's profile called for its use and, interestingly, while conventional lithium did not help her, homeopathic *Lithium* restored her to what she considered nearly her normal self.

Two months after beginning treatment, Sandy reported that her impulsivity had been reduced by 90 percent. As the most telling evidence of this, she could shop "without going crazy." Nail-biting was also no longer a problem and she had gone off caffeine, which she found left her feeling more energetic. In addition, she had lost weight because she was not eating as many carbohydrates.

A month later, Sandy's impulsivity remained improved, but irritability before her period was still a problem, along with other PMS (premenstrual syndrome) symptoms, including fatigue, bloating, tender nipples, and constipation. Dr. Reichenberg-Ullman asked her questions in order to clarify her current symptom picture and learned that Sandy had suffered from serious depression when she was pregnant with each of her children. She described her present sexual interest as "nearly nonexistent." Other new information that emerged was a love of dancing and a craving for chocolate.

Based on this, Dr. Reichenberg-Ullman changed Sandy's remedy to *Sepia* (derived from cuttlefish ink), which was particularly indicated by mood shifts due to hormonal changes. "We generally find success with one homeopathic medicine to treat all of an individual's symptoms," she notes, "however, this was a case where two different medicines in succession were quite beneficial."

At her follow-up consultation two months later, Sandy relayed that her PMS irritability, fatigue, and nipple soreness were much less of a problem, and the rash near her lips had disappeared. Her tendency toward anger was greatly reduced.

After another four months, Dr. Reichenberg-Ullman gave Sandy a higher-potency dose of *Sepia* because her low libido was still distressing her. Four weeks later, she reported that the remedy had worked "miraculously." She credited it with dramatically decreasing her depression.

At a little past a year after the onset of homeopathic treatment, Sandy "continues to feel quite well." Rage is not a problem for her anymore, her PMS is now at a low and manageable level, and mood swings are no longer making her life and marriage miserable. In her case, she is not completely off her medication. At this juncture, she places the percentage of improvement she has experienced as 85 to 90 percent, depending on how much stress she is experiencing.

10 The Shamanic View of Mental Illness

While shamanic practice may seem to be in a completely different category from the other therapies covered in this book, it is actually another holistic medicine that, like acupuncture and homeopathy, addresses disturbances in an individual's electromagnetic or energy field, and in so doing, brings body, mind, and spirit back into alignment. Each of these therapies has its own ways of dealing with energy disturbances, but the goal is the same: the clearing of negative influences and blockages, and the restoration of balance, wholeness, and connectedness.

In addition to its useful analysis of energetic issues, shamanic tradition offers a view of mental disorders that is sorely lacking in the Western world and that holds the key to a whole other way of healing. Disregard of this view has led to treatment based on suppression of symptoms, rather than therapeutic methods that bring the body, mind, and spirit back together. In the shamanic view, mental illness signals "the birth of a healer," explains Malidoma Patrice Somé, Ph.D., an internationally celebrated African shaman, diviner, and teacher. Thus, mental disorders are spiritual emergencies, spiritual crises, and need to be regarded as such to aid the healer in being born.

Shamanic traditions around the globe subscribe to this view, and the West could benefit greatly from absorbing its wisdom. As psychologist and anthropologist Holger Kalweit writes, "If we

What Is Shamanic Healing?

Shamanism is "perhaps the oldest form of practical spirituality in the world, originating in the time of Ice Age people, going back as far as 35,000 B.C."[223] It is also practiced virtually everywhere in the world. A shaman is someone who has gone through advanced initiation into the "hidden" realm. The shaman uses the knowledge gained from the other realm for healing and the good of the community. Shamanic healing is psychic healing, but the term delineates, in particular, indigenous healing that is rooted in traditional ritual.

were able to understand sickness and suffering as processes of physical and psychic transformation, as do Asian peoples and tribal cultures, we would gain a deeper and less biased view of psychosomatic and psychospiritual processes and begin to realize the many opportunities presented by suffering . . . "[224]

What a Shaman Sees in a Mental Hospital

Dr. Somé is a member of the Dagara tribe, which is from an area situated at the intersection of Ghana, the Ivory Coast, and Burkina Faso (formerly Upper Volta) in western Africa. Dr. Somé left his homeland to study in Europe and the United States and holds three master's degrees and two doctorates from the Sorbonne and Brandeis University. He has authored two books, *Ritual: Power, Healing, and Community* and *Of Water and the Spirit.*

The latter is his moving autobiography, which tells of his kidnap at the age of four by Jesuit missionaries who kept him prisoner and trained him as a missionary until at 20 he managed to escape. After an arduous trip back to his village, he underwent an initiation that restored him to his people and opened the way to his shamanic practice. Now dedicated to bringing the healing wisdom of the Dagara tribe to the West, he conducts workshops and classes around the world, while still maintaining a close connection with his village in Burkina Faso.

What those in the West view as mental illness, the Dagara people regard as "good news from the other world." The person going through the crisis has been chosen as a medium for a message to the community that needs to be communicated from the spirit realm. "Mental disorder, behavioral disorder of all kinds, signal the fact that two obviously incompatible energies have merged into the same field," says Dr. Somé. These disturbances result when the person does not get assistance in dealing with the presence of the energy from the spirit realm.

One of the things Dr. Somé encountered when he first came to the United States in 1980 for graduate study was how this country deals with mental illness. When a fellow student was sent to a mental institute due to "nervous depression," Dr. Somé went to visit him.

"I was so shocked. That was the first time I was brought face to face with what is done here to people exhibiting the same symptoms I've seen in my village," says Dr. Somé. What struck him was that the attention given to such symptoms was based on pathology, on the idea that the condition is something that needs to stop. This was in complete opposition to the way his culture views such a situation. As he looked around the stark ward at the patients, some in straitjackets, some zoned out on medications, others screaming, he observed to himself, "So this is how the healers who are attempting to be born are treated in this culture. What a loss! What a loss that a person who is finally being aligned with a power from the other world is just being wasted."

On the ward, Dr. Somé also saw a lot of "beings" hanging around the patients, "entities" that are invisible to most people but that shamans and some psychics are able to see. "They were causing the crisis in these people," he says. It appeared to him that these beings were trying to get the medications and their effects out of the bodies of the people the beings were trying to merge with, and were increasing the patients' pain in the process. "The beings were acting almost like some kind of excavator in the energy field of the people. They were really fierce about that. The people they were doing that to were just screaming and yelling." He couldn't stay in that environment and had to leave.

In the Dagara tradition, the community helps the person reconcile the energies of both worlds—"the world of the spirit that he or she is merged with, and the village and community." That person is able then to serve as a bridge between the worlds and help the living with information and healing they need. Thus, the spiritual crisis ends with the birth of another healer. "The other world's relationship with our world is one of sponsorship," Dr. Somé explains. "More often than not, the knowledge and skills that arise from this kind of merger is a knowledge or a skill that is provided directly from the other world."

> ## In Their Own Words
>
> *"Nobody on Earth escapes life without some form of disability. . . . I prefer to regard bipolar disorder as a 'gift'. . . . In a very real sense, my life has been enriched as a result of my condition."*[225]
>
> —Nancy Rosenfeld, author and bipolar-disorder survivor

The beings who were increasing the pain of the inmates on the mental hospital ward were actually attempting to merge with the inmates in order to get messages through to this world. The people they had chosen to merge with were getting no assistance in learning how to be a bridge between the worlds and the beings' attempts to merge were thwarted. The result was the sustaining of the initial disorder of energy and the aborting of the birth of a healer.

"The Western culture has consistently ignored the birth of the healer," states Dr. Somé. "Consequently, there will be a tendency from the other world to keep trying as many people as possible in an attempt to get somebody's attention. They have to try harder." The spirits are drawn to people whose senses have not been anesthetized. "The sensitivity is pretty much read as an invitation to come in," he notes.

Those who develop so-called mental disorders are those who are sensitive, which is viewed in Western culture as oversensitivity. Indigenous cultures don't see it that way and, as a result, sensitive people don't experience themselves as overly sensitive. In the

171

West, "it is the overload of the culture they're in that is just wrecking them," observes Dr. Somé. The frenetic pace, the bombardment of the senses, and the violent energy that characterize Western culture can overwhelm sensitive people.

The Science of Energy

The foreign energy addressed in shamanic healing enters the energy field that surrounds the body, which is also called the aura. While, unlike shamans, laypeople cannot typically see their aura, they receive evidence of its existence all the time. Have you ever "felt your skin crawl" when you met someone new? Have you ever suddenly and for no apparent reason felt drained or depressed when you walked into a room of people? These reactions are the result of discordant foreign energies entering your energy field, or aura, where they are not a good match with your energy and consequently produce a sense of unease or discomfort.

Energy influences may not be transitory. The energy field around your body is subtle and fragile and can actually be damaged, which renders it more permeable to foreign energies and more likely that they will remain. Among the events or practices that can damage or pollute the aura are emotional or physical trauma, psychic or verbal abuse, other people's negative or bad thoughts about you, and substance abuse. Physicians and psychics alike have noted that the energy field can be occupied by energies that produce mental, emotional, and physical symptoms and, if allowed to remain, can lead to disease.[226]

Psychiatrist Shakuntala Modi, M.D., of Wheeling, West Virginia, has been researching energy field disturbances for over 15 years. She has identified a range of physical and psychological symptoms and conditions that result from such disturbances, including depression, headaches, allergies, uterine disorders, weight gain, stammering, panic disorders, and schizophrenia. Further, under clinical hypnotherapy, 77 out of 100 patients cited foreign "beings" in their aura as responsible for the symptoms or condition for which they were pursuing treatment.

Dr. Modi's research revealed that these beings are "the most common cause of depression" and "the single leading cause of psychiatric problems in general."[227] Dr. Modi also found that after removing the foreign energies from the patient's energy field using hypnotherapy, the patient's symptoms "often cleared up immediately."[228]

The concept of energy disturbances in a person's energy field causing a variety of physical and psychological problems is gaining greater recognition and acceptance in the healing professions and among the public at large. A simple way to look at the issue of "energy pollution" is that, like the environment and your body, your energy field is subject to toxic buildup and requires cleansing to restore it to health. Just as we take measures to clean up our planet and engage in various body detoxification methods such as fasts or colonics, we need to take steps to clear the toxins from our auras.

Shamanic healing is a method for cleansing your energy field of the toxins that are interfering with your physical, emotional, and spiritual health. Or in the case of a being trying to merge with you for healing purposes, shamanic practice brings your energy and that of the being into alignment, thus resolving the symptoms resulting from discordant energy and enabling the healer in you to be born.

Alex: Crazy in the USA, Healer in Africa

To test his belief that the shamanic view of mental illness holds true in the Western world as well as in indigenous cultures, Dr. Somé took a mental patient back to Africa with him, to his village. "I was prompted by my own curiosity to find out whether there's truth in the universality that mental illness could be connected with an alignment with a being from another world," says Dr. Somé.

Alex was an 18-year-old American who had been suffering from psychotic manic-depression for the previous four years. Along with dangerous ups and downs, he had hallucinations and was suicidal. He was in a mental hospital and had been given a lot of drugs, but nothing was helping. "The parents had done everything—unsuccessfully," says Dr. Somé. "They didn't know what else to do."

With their permission, Dr. Somé took their son to Africa. "After eight months there, Alex had become quite normal," Dr.

Somé reports. "He was even able to participate with healers in the business of healing; sitting with them all day long and helping them, assisting them in what they were doing what their clients. . . . He spent about four years in my village." Alex stayed by choice, not because he needed more healing. He felt "much safer in the village than in America."

To bring his energy and that of the being from the spiritual realm into alignment, Alex went through a shamanic ritual designed for that purpose, although it was slightly different from the one used with Dagara people. "He wasn't born in the village, so something else applied. But the result was similar, even though the ritual was not literally the same," explains Dr. Somé. The fact that resonating the energy worked to heal Alex demonstrated to Dr. Somé that the connection between other beings and mental illness is indeed universal.

After the ritual, Alex began to share the messages that the being had for this world. Unfortunately, the people he was talking to didn't speak English (Dr. Somé was away at that point). The whole experience led, however, to Alex going to college to study psychology. He returned to the United States after four years because "he discovered that all the things that he needed to do had been done, and he could then move on with his life."

The last that Dr. Somé heard was that Alex was in graduate school in psychology at Harvard. No one had thought he would ever be able to complete undergraduate studies, much less get an advanced degree.

Dr. Somé sums up what Alex's mental illness was all about: "He was reaching out. It was an emergency call. His job and his purpose was to be a healer. He said no one was paying attention to that."

After seeing how well the shamanic approach worked for Alex, Dr. Somé concluded that beings are just as much an issue in the West as in his community in Africa. "Yet the question still remains, the answer to this problem must be found here, instead of having to go all the way overseas to seek the answer. There has to be a way in which a little bit of attention beyond the pathology of this whole experience leads to the possibility of coming up with the proper ritual to help people."

Bipolar Disorder and Purpose

With bipolar disorder, depression, anxiety, and addiction (the last three epidemic in the United States and the first on the rise), Dr. Somé has found that the main underlying problem is disconnection from one's life purpose. This disconnection "leaves room for some alien energies to come in that don't have anything to do with the kind of promise the person made before coming into this world," the promise of what one will fulfill in one's life. Not fulfilling your promise leaves you subject to "mental" disorders. With this come feelings of uselessness or helplessness, a sense of being "completely adrift in a world without purpose." He believes that 90 percent of the above illnesses have to do with "a perverted purpose, a purpose that has been displaced."

Bipolar disorder in general "has a lot to do with the nature of the contradiction that the person is living," states Dr. Somé. "One pole is the personal promise, the other is the reality. These two poles may not like each other because they're not complementary." The cultural context of the West is often responsible for the contradiction because it doesn't support people in fulfilling their purpose. "They come into a culture that wants them to acquire a certain kind of skill in order to make a living. That messes up a lot of people."

> **With bipolar disorder, Dr. Somé has found that the main underlying problem is disconnection from one's life purpose. This disconnection "leaves room for some alien energies to come in that don't have anything to do with the kind of promise the person made before coming into this world," the promise of what one will fulfill in one's life. Not fulfilling your promise leaves you subject to "mental" disorders.**

The shaman can see what a person's purpose is. "The divination doesn't hide these kinds of things," says Dr. Somé. The shaman's task in this case is to tell people their purpose, but only after preparing them through ritual so they are in a position to understand what is revealed. The ritual used is called a "dupulo," and works to correct the changes done to the original promise. "It's like a disruption of the current path the person is in. It prepares the space for the promise to come alive in the person." After the ritual, the shaman lets a week or two pass, to let it sink in, and then helps the person to become consciously aware of her promise, the specifics of her purpose.

At that point, it is up to them to "take it or leave it," Dr. Somé says. If they decide not to fulfill that purpose, they will go back into illness. The choice is theirs—they can choose to be ill or choose to be aligned with their path.

Dr. Somé gives the example of a man whose promise before being born, the reason why he came into this world, was to work at providing homes for people. "That's a metaphor for a variety of things. One is the actual physical home, another is helping people to feel comfortable with themselves. The man shows up here, finds out how difficult it is, and winds up working in a factory." After receiving the information about his purpose, "he can either start looking into the possibility of being a home builder or a healer who brings stability or groundedness to other people, or not."

Longing for Spiritual Connection

Another common thread that Dr. Somé has noticed in "mental" disorders is "a very ancient ancestral energy that has been placed in stasis, that finally is coming out in the person." His job then is to trace it back, to go back in time to discover what that spirit is. In most cases, the spirit is connected to nature, especially with mountains or big rivers, he says.

In the case of mountains, as an example to explain the phenomenon, "it's a spirit of the mountain that is walking side by side with the person and, as a result, creating a time-space distortion that is affecting the person caught in it." What is needed is a merger or alignment of the two energies, "so the person and the mountain spirit become one." Again, the shaman conducts a specific ritual to bring about this alignment.

Dr. Somé believes that he encounters this situation so often in the United States because "most of the fabric of this country is made up of the energy of the machine, and the result of that is the disconnection and the severing of the past. You can run from the past, but you can't hide from it." The ancestral spirit of the natural world comes visiting. "It's not so much what the spirit wants as it is what the person wants," he says. "The spirit sees in us a call for something grand, something that will make life meaningful, and so the spirit is responding to that."

That call, which we don't even know we are making, reflects "a strong longing for a profound connection, a connection that transcends materialism and possession of things and moves into a tangible cosmic dimension. Most of this longing is unconscious, but for spirits, conscious or unconscious doesn't make any difference." They respond to either.

As part of the ritual to merge the mountain and human energy, those who are receiving the "mountain energy" are sent to a mountain area of their choice, where they pick up a stone that calls to them. They bring that stone back for the rest of the ritual and then keep it as a companion; some even carry it around with them. "The presence of the stone does a lot in tuning the perceptive ability of the person," notes Dr. Somé. "They receive all kinds of information that they can make use of, so it's like they get some tangible guidance from the other world as to how to live their life."

When it is the "river energy," those being called go to the river and, after speaking to the river spirit, find a water stone to bring back for the same kind of ritual as with the mountain spirit.

"People think something extraordinary must be done in an extraordinary situation like this," he says. That's not usually the case. Sometimes it is as simple as carrying a stone.

A Sacred Ritual Approach to Mental Illness

One of the gifts a shaman can bring to the Western world is to help people rediscover ritual, which is so sadly lacking. "The abandonment of ritual can be devastating. From the spiritual viewpoint, ritual is inevitable and necessary if one is to live," Dr. Somé writes in *Ritual: Power, Healing, and Community.* "To say that ritual is needed in the industrialized world is an understatement. We have seen in my own people that it is probably impossible to live a sane life without it."[229]

Dr. Somé did not feel that the rituals from his traditional village could simply be transferred to the West, so over his years of shamanic work here, he has designed rituals that meet the very different needs of this culture. Although the rituals change according to the individual or the group involved, he finds that there is a need for certain rituals in general.

One of these involves helping people discover that their distress is coming from the fact that they are "called by beings from the other world to cooperate with them in doing healing work." Ritual allows them to move out of the distress and accept that calling.

Another ritual need relates to initiation. In indigenous cultures all over the world, young people are initiated into adulthood when they reach a certain age. The lack of such initiation in the West is part of the crisis that people are in here, says Dr. Somé. He urges communities to bring together "the creative juices of people who have had this kind of experience, in an attempt to come up with some kind of an alternative ritual that would at least begin to put a dent in this kind of crisis."

Another ritual that repeatedly speaks to the needs of those coming to him for help entails making a bonfire, and then putting into the bonfire "items that are symbolic of issues carried inside the individuals. . . . It might be the issues of anger and frustration against an ancestor who has left a legacy of murder and enslavement or anything, things that the descendant has to live with," he explains. "If these are approached as things that are blocking the human imagination, the person's life purpose, and even the person's view of life as something that can improve, then it makes sense to begin thinking in terms of how to turn that blockage into a roadway that can lead to something more creative and more fulfilling."

The example of issues with an ancestor touches on rituals designed by Dr. Somé that address a serious dysfunction in Western society and in the process "trigger enlightenment" in participants. These are ancestral rituals, and the dysfunction they are aimed at is the mass turning-of-the-back on ancestors. Some of the spirits trying to come through, as described earlier, may be "ancestors who want to merge with a descendant in an attempt to heal what they weren't able to do while in their physical body."

"Unless the relationship between the living and the dead is in balance, chaos ensues," he says. "The Dagara believe that if such an imbalance exists, it is the duty of the living to heal their ancestors. If these ancestors are not healed, their sick energy will haunt the souls and psyches of those who are responsible for helping them."[230] The rituals focus on healing the relationship with our ancestors, both specific issues of an individual ancestor and the larger cultural issues contained in our past. Dr. Somé has seen extraordinary healing occur at these rituals.

Taking a sacred ritual approach to mental illness rather than regarding the person as a pathological case gives the person affected—and indeed the community at large—the opportunity to begin looking at it from that vantage point too, which leads to a "plethora of opportunities and ritual initiative that can be very, very beneficial to everyone present," states Dr. Somé.

Conclusion

While imbalanced biochemistry may be the central underlying physical feature of bipolar disorder, there are many other factors that combine to produce the particular cluster of symptoms associated with the illness. After all, imbalanced biochemistry can result in a number of disorders. As we have seen, the other four levels of healing—Electromagnetic, Mental, Intuitive, and Spiritual—may be just as implicated as the Physical Level in the development of this particular disorder in a particular person.

Another way to consider bipolar disorder is to explore its deeper message. If you subscribe to the belief that everything in life happens for a purpose, that we are all here to learn and grow as souls, then what is the meaning of bipolar disorder? What is its message for the soul? What does it have to teach? The lessons will, of course, be different for every individual who has bipolar disorder or has a friend, family member, or other loved one with bipolar disorder, but perhaps there are some general themes that run through everyone's experience.

Before we turn to what some of those might be, I want to make it clear that looking for the learning in an illness is not about blaming the victim. Some people have taken the New Age embrace of the ancient idea that every experience has a teaching as license to blame those who are ill for their illnesses, concluding that they must be psychologically messed up or have behaved badly in a past life. This is hardly different from the old, tremendously damaging, and quite false view in the psychiatric profession that "refrigerator" mothers were responsible for their children's mental illnesses.

Looking for the message in illness has nothing to do with blame. It is simply about learning. Every experience in life offers us the opportunity for learning and growth. If we can avail ourselves of that opportunity, every experience has the capacity to make us better people, living our fuller selves, and more completely fulfilling our purpose here on Earth.

So what does bipolar have to teach? A common theme might be learning how to bring balance into one's life. Most of us are trying to achieve this, and it is a challenge amidst the juggling act of modern life, characterized by overstimulation, overscheduling, and overproduction. Bipolar disorder may be an extreme way of teaching moderation and balance, but sometimes that's what it takes. People with bipolar disorder, having faced this challenge to its greatest degree perhaps, are in a unique position to teach others about balance.

Many people with bipolar speak of the guilt, shame, pain, or regret they feel over what they have done in manic states. Perhaps the lesson here is learning how to forgive and love oneself, which naturally leads to greater forgiveness and love of others. Most of us on the planet could learn more about that. Learning that lesson is the center of soul work and truly a gift. Again, people with bipolar disorder have much to teach in this area.

Every illness has the potential to teach those afflicted how to take better care of themselves. While you might think that you are already doing that—by eating a good diet and exercising, for example—illness has a way of highlighting those areas you have neglected. Illness teaches you to attend to body, mind, *and* spirit and shows you the parts of you that are hurting. If you seize this opportunity, you can bring the different levels of yourself into alignment and find your way to a sense of wholeness that brings joy and contentment with it. This kind of happiness is sustaining, in contrast to the high of mania, which is transitory or turns torturous.

If mood is an adaptive mechanism, what do the mood swings of bipolar disorder signify? As discussed in chapter 2, people with bipolar disorder may be less adaptable to change and stress because their regulating mechanisms, which maintain internal homeostasis, are more sensitive than those of people without bipolar and can more easily be thrown off. When considered along with the perspective that mood is an evolutionary adaptation, bipolar disorder may be the proverbial canary in the mine, warning us that "The world is too much with us," as Wordsworth observed.

Perhaps mood disorders are a natural outgrowth of an increasingly toxic, frenetic world, in which mind and spirit receive little attention. Certainly, more people than ever before are suffering from mood disorders. Depression and anxiety disorders are epidemic. In the United States alone, 30 million (1 in 10) people are now on Prozac,[231] and the World Health Organization (WHO) predicts that by the year 2020 depression will be the single leading cause of death around the globe.[232] Perhaps even those who do not have bipolar disorder are losing the ability to adapt to stress and change, and also need to learn how to protect and care for themselves in a new way.

Whatever other message bipolar disorder contains, respect is the message for all—respect for yourself if you have bipolar disorder, and respect from those who don't toward those who do. Although it may not have been their choice, people with bipolar disorder experience the full range of human feeling, often to its furthest reaches. This is a brave way to live, especially when you consider how many people, particularly in the Western world, are doing everything possible not to feel at all. This is not to romanticize the suffering involved in bipolar disorder, but simply to recognize the great strength it requires to live with it.

It is to be hoped that the information in this book enables you to leave the debilitating aspects of bipolar disorder behind and go forward more fully in your life, enriched by the messages you received.

Appendix A

Professional Degrees and Titles

D.C.	Doctor of Chiropractic
D.D.S.	Doctor of Dental Science/Surgery
D.M.D.	Doctor of Dental Medicine
D.O.	Doctor of Osteopathy
D.T.M.&H.	Diploma in Tropical Medicine and Health
H.M.D.	Homeopathic Medical Doctor
L.Ac.	Licensed Acupuncturist
L.C.S.W.	Licensed Clinical Social Worker
M.P.H.	Master of Public Health
M.S.W.	Master of Social Work
N.M.D.	Doctor of Naturopathic Medicine
N.D.	Doctor of Naturopathy

Appendix B

Resources

Practitioners in this book

Lina Garcia, D.D.S., D.M.D.
1443 West Schaumberg Road
Schaumberg, IL 60194
Tel: (847) 985-17777 x39
E-mail: linagarciaj@hotmail.com

Dr. Garcia practices holistic dentistry and holistic healing with a primary modality of osteopathic diagnosis and treatment.

Dietrich Klinghardt, M.D., Ph.D.
1200 112th Avenue NE, Suite A100
Bellevue, WA 98004
Tel: (425) 688-8818

Dr. Klinghardt specializes in Neural Therapy, Applied Psychoneurobiology, and Family Systems Therapy to address energy disturbances and the transgenerational energy legacies at the root of illness.

Devi S. Nambudripad, M.D., D.C., L.Ac., Ph.D.
Pain Clinic
6714 Beach Boulevard
Nambudripad Allergy Research Foundation
6732 Beach Boulevard

Buena Park, CA 90621
Tel: (714) 523-8900
Website: www.naet.com

The Pain Clinic treats various allergy and pain disorders using NAET (Nambudripad's Allergy Elimination Techniques), acupuncture, and chiropractic. The Allergy Research Foundation is a nonprofit organization devoted to conducting clinical trials and studies on NAET and educating the public and professionals alike. Dr. Nambudripad is the author of numerous books, including *Say Goodbye to Illness*.

Judyth Reichenberg-Ullman, N.D., L.C.S.W.
The Northwest Center for Homeopathic Medicine
131 Third Avenue North
Edmonds, WA 98020
Tel: (425) 774-5599
Website: www.healthyhomeopathy.com

In practice with her husband, Robert Ullman, Dr. Reichenberg-Ullman is a licensed naturopathic physician board certified in homeopathy. She has been practicing for 18 years and is the author/co-author of six books on homeopathic medicine, including *Prozac-Free, Ritalin-Free Kids,* and *Whole Woman Homeopathy*.

Julia Ross, M.A.
Recovery Systems
147 Lomita Drive, Suite D
Mill Valley, CA 94941
Tel: (415) 383-3611 x2
Website: www.dietcure.com

Ross, a pioneer in nutritional psychology and author of *The Mood Cure* and *The Diet Cure,* has 25 years of experience directing programs that address mood problems, addiction, and eating disorders. Recovery Systems provides psychological/nutritional assessment and ongoing nutritional counseling.

Malidoma Patrice Somé, Ph.D.
236 West East Avenue, Suite A, PMB 199
Chico, CA 95926
Tel: (530) 894-0740
E-mail: rowenap@jps.net (Rowena Pantaleon, Dr. Somé's assistant)
Website: www.malidoma.com and www.villagewisdom.net

Dr. Somé is an African shaman, diviner, and teacher who brings the healing wisdom of the Dagara tribe to the West.

William J. Walsh, Ph.D.
Health Research Institute and Pfeiffer Treatment Center
4575 Weaver Parkway
Warrenville, IL 60555
Tel: (630) 505-0300
E-mail: info@hriptc.org
Website: www.hriptc.org

Chief scientist/biochemical researcher at HRI-PTC, a nonprofit organization based in Illinois, with services in Minnesota, Maryland, Arizona, and California; outpatient clinic with collaboration between medical doctors, biochemists, and nutritionists, offering individualized nutrient therapy for bipolar disorder, autism, ADD, depression, schizophrenia, and other conditions.

Bradford S. Weeks, M.D.
P.O. Box 740
Clinton, WA 98236
Tel: (360) 341-2303
E-mail: admin@weeksmd.com
Website: www.weeksmd.com

Dr. Weeks' medical and psychiatric orientation is biological and biochemical, with a particular focus on Anthroposophic medicine. Among the therapeutic modalities he employs in this context are targeted nutritional therapies, IV therapies for detoxification and replenishment, apitherapy (bee venom therapy), and Psychology of Mind. In his practice, he treats people with dis-ease of all kinds, from "mental" disorders to severe degenerative physical disorders such as multiple sclerosis, arthritis, immune dysfunction, cardiac disease, and cancer. He always looks for the reasons that the patient feels they are ill and how the patient wants to change things once wellness is reclaimed. A favorite question for patients is: What are you doing with your creative energy?

Endnotes

Introduction

1. C. J. L. Murray, and A. D. Lopez, eds., *Summary: The Global Burden of Disease: A Comprehensive Assessment of Mortality and Disability from Diseases, Injuries, and Risk Factors in 1990 and Projected to 2020* (Cambridge: Harvard School of Public Health on Behalf of the World Health Organization and the World Bank, Harvard University Press, 1996). Available on the Internet at: http://www.who.int/msa/mnh/ems/dalys/intro.htm. Cited in U.S. Department of Health and Human Services, "Mental Health: A Report of the Surgeon General, Executive Summary," (Rockville, Md.: U.S. Department of Health and Human Services, Substance Abuse and Mental Health Services Administration, Center for Mental Health Services, National Institutes of Health, National Institute of Mental Health, 1999): ix.

2. C. J. L. Murray, and A. D. Lopez, eds., *Summary: The Global Burden of Disease: A Comprehensive Assessment of Mortality and Disability from Diseases, Injuries, and Risk Factors in 1990 and Projected to 2020* (Cambridge: Harvard School of Public Health on Behalf of the World Health Organization and the World Bank, Harvard University Press, 1996). Available on the Internet at: http://www.who.int/msa/mnh/ems/dalys/intro.htm.

3. R. C. Kessler, et al., "A Methodology for Estimating the 12-Month Prevalence of Serious Mental Illness," in: R. W. Manderscheid and M. J. Henderson, eds., *Mental Health, United States, 1999* (Rockville, Md.: Center for Mental Health Services, 1998): 99–109.

4. Center for Mental Health Services, *Survey of Mental Health Organizations and General Mental Health Services* (Rockville, Md.: Center for Mental Health Services, 1998).

5. 1990 is the most recent year for which estimates are available, according to "Mental Health: A Report of the U.S. Surgeon General" (1999);

189

available on the Internet at http://www.surgeongeneral.gov/library/mental-health/chapter6/sec2.html#figure6_3. D. P. Rice and L. S. Miller, "The Economic Burden of Schizophrenia: Conceptual and Methodological Issues, and Cost Estimates," in M. Moscarelli, A. Rupp, and N. Sartorious, eds., *Handbook of Mental Health Economics and Health Policy: Schizophrenia,* Vol. 1 (New York: John Wiley and Sons, 1996): 321–4.

6. The full text of the letter is available on the Internet at: http://www.connix.com/~narpa/mosher.htm

1: What Is Bipolar Disorder and Who Suffers from It?

7. Kay Redfield Jamison, *An Unquiet Mind: A Memoir of Moods and Madness* (New York: Knopf, 1995): 182.

8. Patty Duke and Gloria Hochman, *A Brilliant Madness: Living with Manic-Depressive Illness* (New York: Bantam, 1993): 49.

9. Demitri Papolos, M.D., and Janice Papolos, *Overcoming Depression: The Definitive Resource for Patients and Families Who Live with Depression and Manic-Depression* (New York: HarperPerennial, 1997): 10.

10. The sources for the statistics are: Francis Mark Mondimore, M.D., *Bipolar Disorder: A Guide for Patients and Families* (Baltimore: Johns Hopkins University Press, 1999): ix. Jeffrey Kluger with Sora Song, "Young and Bipolar," *Time* (August 19, 2002, cover story). Kay Redfield Jamison, "Manic-Depressive Illness and Creativity," *Scientific American* (February 1995): 64. NARSAD, "Fact Sheet: The Treatment of Bipolar Disorder," National Alliance for Research on Schizophrenia and Depression (NARSAD), 60 Cutter Mill Road, Suite 404, Great Neck, NY 11021; tel: (516) 829-0092 or (800) 829-8289; website: www.narsad.org.

11. National DMDA, "Consumer's Guide to Depression and Manic Depression," National DMDA (Depressive and Manic-Depressive Association), 730 North Franklin Street, Suite 501, Chicago, IL 60610-3526; tel: (800) 826-3632 or (312) 642-0049; website: www.ndmda.org.

12. Source: Jeffrey Kluger with Sora Song, "Young and Bipolar," *Time* (August 19, 2002, cover story).

13. David A. Kahn, M.D., et al., "Treatment of Bipolar Disorder: A Guide for Patients and Families," A Postgraduate Medicine Special Report, April 2000; available from NDMDA (National Depressive and Manic-Depressive Association), tel: 800-826-3632, website: www.ndmda.org; or NAMI (National Alliance for the Mentally Ill), tel: 800-950-6264, website: www.nami.org.

14. D. A. Reger, M. E. Farm, and D. S. Rae, "Comorbidity of Mental Disorders with Alcohol and Other Drug Abuse: Results from the

Epidemiologic Catchment Area Study," *Journal of the American Medical Association* 264 (1990): 2511–8.

15. Demitri Papolos, M.D., and Janice Papolos, *Overcoming Depression: The Definitive Resource for Patients and Families Who Live with Depression and Manic-Depression* (New York: HarperPerennial, 1997): 248.

16. NARSAD, "Fact Sheet: The Warning Signs of Suicide," NARSAD (National Alliance for Research on Schizophrenia and Depression), 60 Cutter Mill Road, Suite 404, Great Neck, NY 11021; tel: (516) 829-0091; fax: (516) 487-6930; website: www.narsad.org.

17. David A. Kahn, M.D., et al., "Treatment of Bipolar Disorder: A Guide for Patients and Families," A Postgraduate Medicine Special Report, April 2000; available from NDMDA (National Depressive and Manic-Depressive Association), tel: 800-826-3632, website: www.ndmda.org; or NAMI (National Alliance for the Mentally Ill), tel: 800-950-6264, website: www.nami.org.

18. NAMI, "Understanding Major Depression," NAMI (National Alliance for the Mentally Ill), Colonial Place Three, 2107 Wilson Blvd., Suite 300, Alexandria, VA 22201-3042; tel: (888) 999-NAMI (6264) or (703) 524-7600; website: www.nami.org.

19. NARSAD, "Fact Sheet: The Warning Signs of Suicide," NARSAD (National Alliance for Research on Schizophrenia and Depression), 60 Cutter Mill Road, Suite 404, Great Neck, NY 11021; tel: (516) 829-0091; fax: (516) 487-6930; website: www.narsad.org.

20. Jeffrey Kluger with Sora Song, "Young and Bipolar," *Time* (August 19, 2002, cover story).

21. Rita Elkins, *Depression and Natural Medicine: A Nutritional Approach to Depression and Mood Swings* (Pleasant Grove, Utah: Woodland Publishing, 1995): 16. Demitri Papolos, M.D., and Janice Papolos, *Overcoming Depression: The Definitive Resource for Patients and Families Who Live with Depression and Manic-Depression* (New York: HarperPerennial, 1997): 270.

22. American Psychiatric Association, *DSM-IV-TR* (*Diagnostic and Statistical Manual of Mental Disorders, 4th Edition, Text Revision*), Washington, D.C.: American Psychiatric Association, 2000: 382–3.

23. Ibid., 345–401.

24. *DSM-IV-TR,* 386.

25. *DSM-IV-TR,* 362.

26. *DSM-IV-TR,* 356.

27. *DSM-IV-TR,* 394.

28. *DSM-IV-TR,* 397.

29. *DSM-IV-TR,* 362.

30. Kay Redfield Jamison, *An Unquiet Mind: A Memoir of Moods and Madness* (New York: Knopf, 1995): 45.

31. Francis Mark Mondimore, M.D., *Bipolar Disorder: A Guide for Patients and Families* (Baltimore: Johns Hopkins University Press, 1999): 51.

32. Patty Duke and Gloria Hochman, *A Brilliant Madness: Living with Manic-Depressive Illness* (New York: Bantam, 1993): 1.

33. Kay Redfield Jamison, *Touched with Fire: Manic-Depressive Illness and the Artistic Temperament,* (New York: Free Press/Simon & Schuster, 1993): 103.

34. Kay Redfield Jamison, "Manic-Depressive Illness and Creativity," *Scientific American* (February 1995): 66.

35. Ibid., 65.

36. Kay Redfield Jamison, *Touched with Fire: Manic-Depressive Illness and the Artistic Temperament,* (New York: Free Press/Simon & Schuster, 1993): 249.

37. Ibid., 243.

38. Ibid., 103.

39. Francis Mark Mondimore, M.D., *Bipolar Disorder: A Guide for Patients and Families* (Baltimore: Johns Hopkins University Press, 1999): 214.

40. Patty Duke and Gloria Hochman, *A Brilliant Madness: Living with Manic-Depressive Illness* (New York: Bantam, 1993): 203–209. Kay Redfield Jamison, *Touched with Fire: Manic-Depressive Illness and the Artistic Temperament,* (New York: Free Press/Simon & Schuster, 1993). Francis Mark Mondimore, M.D., *Bipolar Disorder: A Guide for Patients and Families* (Baltimore: Johns Hopkins University Press, 1999): ix.

41. Demitri Papolos, M.D., and Janice Papolos, *Overcoming Depression: The Definitive Resource for Patients and Families Who Live with Depression and Manic-Depression* (New York: HarperPerennial, 1997): 32.

42. Quoted in Francis Mark Mondimore, M.D., *Bipolar Disorder: A Guide for Patients and Families* (Baltimore: Johns Hopkins University Press, 1999): 62.

43. Demitri Papolos, M.D., and Janice Papolos, *Overcoming Depression: The Definitive Resource for Patients and Families Who Live with Depression and Manic-Depression* (New York: HarperPerennial, 1997): 10. Peter C. Whybrow, M.D., *A Mood Apart: The Thinker's Guide to Emotion and Its Disorders* (New York: HarperPerennial, 1997): 255.

44. Peter C. Whybrow, M.D., *A Mood Apart: The Thinker's Guide to Emotion and Its Disorders* (New York: HarperPerennial, 1997): 255.

45. Stanley W. Jackson, *Melancholia and Depression, from Hippocratic Times to Modern Times* (New Haven: Yale University Press, 1986): 253–4.

46. Lewis Wolpert, *Malignant Sadness: The Anatomy of Depression* (New York: The Free Press, 1999): 3–4.

47. Francis Mark Mondimore, M.D., *Bipolar Disorder: A Guide for Patients and Families* (Baltimore: Johns Hopkins University Press, 1999): 62–3.

48. Demitri Papolos, M.D., and Janice Papolos, *Overcoming Depression: The Definitive Resource for Patients and Families Who Live with Depression and Manic-Depression* (New York: HarperPerennial, 1997): 32–3.

49. Catherine Carrigan, *Healing Depression: A Holistic Guide* (New York: Marlowe and Company, 2000): 75.

50. Joseph Glenmullen, M.D., *Prozac Backlash* (New York: Touchstone/Simon & Schuster, 2000): 16.

51. E. C. Azmitia and P. M. Whitaker-Azmitia, "Awakening the sleeping giant: anatomy and plasticity of the brain serotonergic system," *Journal of Clinical Psychiatry* 52:12 suppl. (1991): 4–16. Cited in Joseph Glenmullen, M.D., *Prozac Backlash* (New York: Touchstone/Simon & Schuster, 2000): 16.

52. Peter C. Whybrow, M.D., *A Mood Apart: The Thinker's Guide to Emotion and Its Disorders* (New York: HarperPerennial, 1997): 46.

53. Ibid., 205.

54. Joseph Glenmullen, M.D., *Prozac Backlash* (New York: Touchstone/Simon & Schuster, 2000): 340.

55. *Taber's Cyclopedic Medical Dictionary*, 17th ed. (Philadelphia: F. A. Davis Company, 1993): 662, 1318.

56. Peter R. Breggin, M.D., and David Cohen, Ph.D., *Your Drug May Be Your Problem: How and Why to Stop Taking Psychiatric Medications* (Reading, Mass.: Perseus Books, 1999): 36.

57. Jeffrey Kluger with Sora Song, "Young and Bipolar," *Time* (August 19, 2002, cover story).

58. Peter R. Breggin, M.D., and David Cohen, Ph.D., *Your Drug May Be Your Problem: How and Why to Stop Taking Psychiatric Medications* (Reading, Mass.: Perseus Books, 1999): 63.

59. C. B. Nemeroff, "An Ever-Increasing Pharmacopoeia for the Management of Patients with Bipolar Disorder," *Journal of Clinical Psychiatry* 61: suppl. 13 (2000): 19–25.

60. Peter R. Breggin, M.D., and David Cohen, Ph.D., *Your Drug May*

Be Your Problem: How and Why to Stop Taking Psychiatric Medications (Reading, Mass.: Perseus Books, 1999): 75.

61. Ibid., 76–7.

62. Ibid., 78.

63. Joseph Glenmullen, M.D., *Prozac Backlash* (New York: Touchstone/Simon & Schuster, 2000): 16.

64. Michael T. Murray, N.D., *Natural Alternatives to Prozac* (New York: Quill/William Morrow, 1996): 4.

65. Ibid., 2.

66. Ibid.

67. Maryann Napoli, "A New Assessment of Depression Drugs," *HealthFacts* 24:7 (July 31, 1999): 4.

68. Harvard Medical School, "Update on Mood Disorders: Part II," *Harvard Mental Health Letter* 11:7 (1995): 3.

69. "Depression Drugs Widely Prescribed to Children," *Health Watch* 4:2 (June 30, 1999): 2.

70. A. C. Pande and M. E. Sayler, "Adverse Events and Treatment Discontinuations in Fluoxetine Clinical Trials," *International Journal of Psychopharmacology* 8 (1993): 267–9.

71. Peter R. Breggin, M.D., and David Cohen, Ph.D., *Your Drug May Be Your Problem: How and Why to Stop Taking Psychiatric Medications* (Reading, Mass.: Perseus Books, 1999): 68.

72. Joseph Glenmullen, M.D., *Prozac Backlash* (New York: Touchstone/Simon & Schuster, 2000). Peter R. Breggin, M.D., and David Cohen, Ph.D., *Your Drug May Be Your Problem: How and Why to Stop Taking Psychiatric Medications* (Reading, Mass.: Perseus Books, 1999): 46–7.

73. Francis Mark Mondimore, M.D., *Bipolar Disorder: A Guide for Patients and Families* (Baltimore: Johns Hopkins University Press, 1999): 107.

74. Anne Harding, "Antidepressants Hazardous for Some Mentally Ill," Reuters Health Information (March 20, 2001); available on the Internet at http://www.nlm.nih.gov/medlineplus/news/fullstory_832.html

2: Causes, Triggers, and Contributors

75. Quoted on the website of Volunteers In Psychotherapy, in an article entitled "Are Personal and Emotional Problems Diseases?" available on the Internet at www.ctvip.org/weB2c.html, or contact Richard Shulman, Ph.D., Director, Volunteers In Psychotherapy, Inc., 7 South Main Street, West Hartford, CT 06107; tel: (860) 233-5115.

76. Ibid.

77. Ibid.

78. Joseph Glenmullen, M.D., *Prozac Backlash* (New York: Touchstone/Simon & Schuster, 2000): 193.

79. U.S. Department of Health and Human Services, "Mental Health: A Report of the Surgeon General, Executive Summary," (Rockville, Md.: U.S. Department of Health and Human Services, Substance Abuse and Mental Health Services Administration, Center for Mental Health Services, National Institutes of Health, National Institute of Mental Health, 1999): x.

80. Joseph Glenmullen, M.D., *Prozac Backlash* (New York: Touchstone/Simon & Schuster, 2000): 198.

81. Jeffrey Kluger with Sora Song, "Young and Bipolar," *Time* (August 19, 2002, cover story).

82. Ibid.

83. Peter C. Whybrow, M.D., *A Mood Apart: The Thinker's Guide to Emotion and Its Disorders* (New York: HarperPerennial, 1997): 152, 163, 165.

84. Francis Mark Mondimore, M.D., *Bipolar Disorder: A Guide for Patients and Families* (Baltimore: Johns Hopkins University Press, 1999): 225.

85. Richard Leviton, *The Healthy Living Space* (Charlottesville, Va.: Hampton Roads, 2001): 2.

86. Ibid., 3.

87. "Doctors Warn Developmental Disabilities Epidemic from Toxins," *LDA (Learning Disabilities Association of America) Newsbriefs* 35:4 (July/August 2000): 3–5; executive summary from the report by the Greater Boston Physicians for Social Responsibility, *In Harm's Way—Toxic Threats to Child Development*, available at http://www.igc.org/psr/ihw.htm; for LDA, http://www.ldanatl.org.

88. Philip J. Landrigan, *Environmental Neurotoxicology* (Washington, D.C.: National Academy Press, 1992): 2; cited in Richard Leviton, *The Healthy Living Space* (Charlottesville, Va.: Hampton Roads, 2001): 13.

89. Cited in: Syd Baumel, *Dealing with Depression Naturally* (Los Angeles: Keats Publishing, 2000): 31.

90. Sherry A. Rogers, M.D., *Depression—Cured at Last!* (Sarasota: SK Publishing, 1997): 94.

91. John Foster, M.D., "Is Depression Natural in an Unnatural World?" *Well-Being Journal* (Spring 2001): 11; website: www.wellbeingjournal.com.

92. Catherine Carrigan, *Healing Depression: A Holistic Guide* (New York: Marlowe and Company, 2000): 62.

93. Dietrich Klinghardt, M.D., Ph.D., "Amalgam/Mercury Detox as a Treatment for Chronic Viral, Bacterial, and Fungal Illnesses," lecture presented at the Annual Meeting of the International and American Academy of Clinical Nutrition, San Diego, Calif., September 1996.

94. Morton Walker, D.P.M., *Elements of Danger: Protect Yourself Against the Hazards of Modern Dentistry* (Charlottesville, Va.: Hampton Roads, 2000): 138, 141.

95. Ibid., 144–5.

96. Syd Baumel, *Dealing with Depression Naturally* (Los Angeles: Keats Publishing, 2000): 34.

97. Ibid., 35.

98. W. D. Kaehny, et al., "Gastrointestinal Absorption of Aluminum from Aluminum-Containing Antacids," *New England Journal of Medicine* 296 (1977): 1389–90. D. P. Perl and A. R. Bordy, "Detection of Aluminum by Semi-X-Ray Spectrometry with Neurofibrillary Tangle-Bearing Neurons of Alzheimer's Disease," *Neurotox* (1990): 133–7. Morton Walker, D.P.M., *Elements of Danger: Protect Yourself Against the Hazards of Modern Dentistry* (Charlottesville, Va.: Hampton Roads, 2000): 218–9.

99. Rita Elkins, *Depression and Natural Medicine: A Nutritional Approach to Depression and Mood Swings* (Pleasant Grove, Utah: Woodland Publishing, 1995): 117.

100. Sherry A. Rogers, M.D., *Depression—Cured at Last!* (Sarasota: SK Publishing, 1997): 460.

101. Ibid., 461–2.

102. Ibid., 165–7.

103. Ibid., 166.

104. Personal communication, 2001.

105. John N. Hathcock, *Nutritional Toxicology,* Vol. I (New York: Academic Press, 1982): 462. L. D. Stegink and L. J. Filer Jr., eds., *Aspartame* (New York: Marcel Dekker, 1984): 350, 359. Bryan Ballantyne, Timothy Marrs, and Paul Turner, eds., *General and Applied Toxicology,* Vol. 1 (New York: Stockton Press, 1993): 482.

106. Hyman J. Roberts, "Reactions Attributed to Aspartame Containing Products: 551 Cases," *Natural Food & Farming* (March 1992): 23–8.

107. Leon Chaitow, *Thorson's Guide to Amino Acids* (London: Thorson, 1991): 95.

108. Susan C. Smolinske, *Handbook of Food, Drug, and Cosmetic Excipients* (Boca Raton: CRC Press, 1992): 236.

109. Bernard Rimland, Ph.D., "The Feingold Diet: An Assessment of the Reviews by Marttes, by Kavale and Forness and Others," *Journal of*

Learning Disabilities 16:6 (June/July 1983): 331. (Available from the Autism Research Institute, Publication #51.)

110. Richard A. Kunin, M.D., "Principles That Identify Orthomolecular Medicine: A Unique Medical Specialty," available on the Internet at: http://www.orthomed.org/kunin.htm.

111. Claudio Galli and Artemis P. Simopoulos, ed., *Dietary W3 and W6 Fatty Acids: Biological Effects and Nutritional Essentiality* (New York: Kluwer/Plenum, 1989). Claudio Galli and Artemis P. Simopoulos, *Effects of Fatty Acids and Lipids in Health and Disease*, New York: S. Karger, 1994. Joseph Mercola, "Where's the Real Beef?" available on the Internet at www.mercola.com/beef/main.htm.

112. Presenter statement by Andrew Stoll, M.D., in the DAN! (Defeat Autism Now!) 2000 Conference booklet: 8; published by the Autism Research Institute in San Diego, Calif. (fax: 619-563-6840 or website: www.autism.com/ari).

113. M. A. Crawford, A. G. Hassam, and P. A. Stevens, "Essential Fatty Acid Requirements in Pregnancy and Lactation with Special Reference to Brain Development," *Prog Lipid Res* 20 (1981): 31–40.

114. "Healing Mood Disorders with Essential Fatty Acids," *Doctors' Prescription for Healthy Living* 4:6, 1.

115. "Researchers Discover Five Good-Mood Foods," *Today's Chiropractic* 28:2 (April 30, 1999): 26.

116. Rhian Edwards, et al., "Omega-3 polyunsaturated fatty acid levels in the diet and in red blood cell membranes of depressed patients," *Journal of Affective Disorders* 48 (1998): 149-55. Peter B. Adams, et al., "Arachidonic Acid to Eicosapentaenoic Acid Ratio in Blood Correlates Positively with Symptoms of Depression," *Lipids* 31: suppl. (1996): S157–61.

117. Barbara S. Levine. "Most Frequently Asked Questions about DHA," *Nutrition Today* 32 (November/December 1997): 248–9.

118. Eva Edelman, *Natural Healing for Schizophrenia and Other Common Mental Disorders*, 3d ed. (Eugene, Ore.: Borage Books, 2001): 62.

119. Kristen A. Bruinsma and Douglas L. Taren, "Dieting, Essential Fatty Acid Intake, and Depression," *Nutrition Reviews* 58 (April 2000): 98–108.

120. Joseph R. Hibbeln, "Fish Consumption and Major Depression," *The Lancet* 351 (April 18, 1998): 1213.

121. Eva Edelman, *Natural Healing for Schizophrenia and Other Common Mental Disorders*, 3d ed. (Eugene, Ore.: Borage Books, 2001): 143.

G. Chouinard, et al., "Tryptophan in the Treatment of Depression and Mania," *Adv Biol Psychiatry* 10 (1983): 47–66. G. Chouinard, et al., "A Controlled Clinical Trial of L-Tryptophan in Acute Mania," *Biol Psychiatry* 20 (1985): 546–7.

122. Prevention's *New Encyclopedia of Common Diseases* (Emmaus, Pa.: Rodale Press, 1985): 230.

123. H. Beckman, "Phenylalanine in Affective Disorders," *Adv Biol Psychiatry* 10 (1983): 137–47. C. Gibson and A. Gelenberg, "Tyrosine for Depression," *Adv Biol Psychiatry* 10 (1983): 148–59.

124. Eva Edelman, *Natural Healing for Schizophrenia and Other Common Mental Disorders*, 3d ed. (Eugene, Ore.: Borage Books, 2001): 144.

125. B. M. Cohen, et al., "Lecithin in the Treatment of Mania," *American Journal of Psychiatry* 139 (1982): 1162–4. A. L. Stoll, et al., "Choline in the Treatment of Rapid-Cycling Bipolar Disorder: Clinical and Neurochemical Findings in Lithium-Treated Patients," *Bio Psychiatry* 40:5 (September 1, 1996): 382–8. R. S. Jope, et al., "The Phosphoinositide Signal Transduction System is Impaired in Bipolar Affective Disorder Brain," *J Neurochem* 66:6 (June 1996): 2402–9.

126. Eva Edelman, *Natural Healing for Schizophrenia and Other Common Mental Disorders*, 3d ed. (Eugene, Ore.: Borage Books, 2001): 134.

127. E. H. Cook and B. L. Leventhal, "The Serotonin System in Autism," *Curr Opin Pediatr* 8:4 (August 1996): 348–54.

128. Syd Baumel, *Dealing with Depression Naturally* (Los Angeles: Keats Publishing, 2000): 12.

129. Ronald Hoffman, "Beyond Prozac: Natural Therapies for Anxiety and Depression," *Innovation: The Health Letter of FAIM* (January 31, 1999): 10–11, 13, 15, 17, 19.

130. Peter C. Whybrow, M.D., *A Mood Apart: The Thinker's Guide to Emotion and Its Disorders* (New York: HarperPerennial, 1997): 212.

131. Francis Mark Mondimore, M.D., *Bipolar Disorder: A Guide for Patients and Families* (Baltimore: Johns Hopkins University Press, 1999): 203.

132. Demitri Papolos, M.D., and Janice Papolos, *Overcoming Depression: The Definitive Resource for Patients and Families Who Live with Depression and Manic-Depression* (New York: HarperPerennial, 1997): 93.

133. Peter R. Breggin, M.D., and David Cohen, Ph.D., *Your Drug May Be Your Problem: How and Why to Stop Taking Psychiatric Medications* (Reading, Mass.: Perseus Books, 1999): 75.

134. Sherry A. Rogers, M.D., *Depression—Cured at Last!* (Sarasota: SK Publishing, 1997): 408–10.

135. Peter C. Whybrow, M.D., *A Mood Apart: The Thinker's Guide to Emotion and Its Disorders* (New York: HarperPerennial, 1997): 165–6.

136. Burton Goldberg and the editors of *Alternative Medicine, Women's Health Series: 2* (Tiburon: Future Medicine Publishing, 1998): 208–9.

137. John R. Lee, M.D., *What Your Doctor May Not Tell You About Menopause* (New York: Warner Books, 1996): 103, 229.

138. Sherry A. Rogers, M.D., *Depression—Cured at Last!* (Sarasota: SK Publishing, 1997): 403.

139. Peter C. Whybrow, M.D., *A Mood Apart: The Thinker's Guide to Emotion and Its Disorders* (New York: HarperPerennial, 1997): 202.

140. Michael Lesser, M.D., *Nutrition and Vitamin Therapy* (New York: Bantam, 1981): 171.

141. William J. Walsh, Ph.D., "The Critical role of Nutrients in Severe Mental Symptoms," Available on the Internet (www.alternativemental health.com/articles/article-pffeiffer.htm).

142. American Psychiatric Association, *DSM-IV-TR* (*Diagnostic and Statistical Manual of Mental Disorders, 4th Edition, Text Revision*) (Washington, D.C.: American Psychiatric Association, 2000): 403.

143. E. Fuller Torrey, et al., "Birth Seasonality in Bipolar Disorder, Schizophrenia, Schizoaffective Disorder, and Stillbirths," *Schizophrenia Research* 21 (1996): 141–9.

144. *DSM-IV-TR*, 407.

145. Michael T. Murray, N.D., *Natural Alternatives to Prozac* (New York: Quill/William Morrow, 1996): 56. Sherry A. Rogers, M.D., *Depression—Cured at Last!* (Sarasota: SK Publishing, 1997): 144–5.

146. Joseph Glenmullen, M.D., *Prozac Backlash* (New York: Touchstone/Simon & Schuster, 2000): 87.

147. Ibid., 86.

148. Patty Duke and Gloria Hochman, *A Brilliant Madness: Living with Manic-Depressive Illness* (New York: Bantam, 1993): 9.

149. Ibid., xx.

150. Rita Elkins, *Depression and Natural Medicine: A Nutritional Approach to Depression and Mood Swings* (Pleasant Grove, Utah: Woodland Publishing, 1995): 138.

151. Ibid.

152. Rita Elkins, *Depression and Natural Medicine: A Nutritional Approach to Depression and Mood Swings* (Pleasant Grove, Utah:

Woodland Publishing, 1995): 138. Eva Edelman, *Natural Healing for Schizophrenia and Other Common Mental Disorders*, 3d ed. (Eugene, Ore.: Borage Books, 2001): 85.

153. Peter C. Whybrow, M.D., *A Mood Apart: The Thinker's Guide to Emotion and Its Disorders* (New York: HarperPerennial, 1997): 213.

154. Eva Edelman, *Natural Healing for Schizophrenia and Other Common Mental Disorders*, 3d ed. (Eugene, Ore.: Borage Books, 2001): 86.

155. Peter C. Whybrow, M.D., *A Mood Apart: The Thinker's Guide to Emotion and Its Disorders* (New York: HarperPerennial, 1997): 162. Francis Mark Mondimore, M.D., *Bipolar Disorder: A Guide for Patients and Families* (Baltimore: Johns Hopkins University Press, 1999): 190.

156. Demitri Papolos, M.D., and Janice Papolos, *Overcoming Depression: The Definitive Resource for Patients and Families Who Live with Depression and Manic-Depression* (New York: HarperPerennial, 1997): 211–2.

157. Peter C. Whybrow, M.D., *A Mood Apart: The Thinker's Guide to Emotion and Its Disorders* (New York: HarperPerennial, 1997): 250.

158. Rita Elkins, *Depression and Natural Medicine: A Nutritional Approach to Depression and Mood Swings* (Pleasant Grove, Utah: Woodland Publishing, 1995): 103. Eva Edelman, *Natural Healing for Schizophrenia and Other Common Mental Disorders*, 3d ed. (Eugene, Ore.: Borage Books, 2001): 40.

159. Amy Norton, "Exercise Beats Drugs for Some with Depression," Reuters Health Information (March 28, 2001); available on the Internet at: http://www.nlm.nih.gov/medlineplus/news/fullstory_949.html.

160. Rita Elkins, *Depression and Natural Medicine: A Nutritional Approach to Depression and Mood Swings* (Pleasant Grove, Utah: Woodland Publishing, 1995): 103.

161. Eva Edelman, *Natural Healing for Schizophrenia and Other Common Mental Disorders*, 3d ed. (Eugene, Ore.: Borage Books, 2001): 134.

162. Ibid., 40.

163. Peter C. Whybrow, M.D., *A Mood Apart: The Thinker's Guide to Emotion and Its Disorders* (New York: HarperPerennial, 1997): 158, 162.

164. Ibid., 162.

165. Jan Fawcett, M.D., Bernard Golden, Ph.D., and Nancy Rosenfeld, *New Hope for People with Bipolar Disorder* (Roseville, Calif.: Prima, 2000): 26.

166. Patty Duke and Gloria Hochman, *A Brilliant Madness: Living with Manic-Depressive Illness* (New York: Bantam, 1993): 123.

167. Demitri Papolos, M.D., and Janice Papolos, *Overcoming Depression: The Definitive Resource for Patients and Families Who Live with Depression and Manic-Depression* (New York: HarperPerennial, 1997): 190.

168. Peter C. Whybrow, M.D., *A Mood Apart: The Thinker's Guide to Emotion and Its Disorders* (New York: HarperPerennial, 1997): 250.

3: A Model for Healing

169. Quoted in Jeffrey Kluger with Sora Song, "Young and Bipolar," *Time* (August 19, 2002, cover story).

170. Richard Leviton, "Migraines, Seizures, and Mercury Toxicity," *Alternative Medicine Digest* 21 (December 1997/January 1998): 61.

4: Healing from a Cellular to a Spiritual Level: Biological Medicine

171. Bradford S. Weeks, M.D., "The Role of Essential Fatty Acids in Mental Health," Lecture to the Well Mind Association, Seattle, Washington, October 2001.

172. From *Mood Disorders: Toward a New Psychobiology,* by Drs. Peter Whybrow, Hagop Akiskal, and William McKinney, quoted in Demitri Papolos, M.D., and Janice Papolos, *Overcoming Depression: The Definitive Resource for Patients and Families Who Live with Depression and Manic-Depression* (New York: HarperPerennial, 1997): 25–6.

173. The FDA has made it illegal to market GHB in the United States. Many physicians, having witnessed its effectiveness as a sleep aid and antianxiety agent, among other medical applications, maintain that the banning of this highly useful supplement is politically motivated. See: Steven Wm. Fowkes, "GHB Report to the California Legislature," available on the Internet at: http://www.ceri.com/report.htm.

Chapter 5: Biochemical Treatment of Bipolar Disorder

174. William J. Walsh, Ph.D., "Biochemical Treatment: Medicines for the Next Century," *NOHA (Nutrition for Optimal Health Association) News* 16:3 (Summer 1991), available on the HRI-PTC Website (www.hriptc.org/nextcentury.htm).

175. From the film *Masks of Madness: Science of Healing,* written, produced, and directed by Connie Bortnick, produced in associated with the Canadian Schizophrenia Foundation, 16 Florence Avenue, Toronto, Ontario M2N 1E9 Canada (Sisyphus Communications, Ltd., 1998). To contact the Institute for Optimum Nutrition (ION), Blades Court, Deodar Road, London SW15 2NU England; tel: 020 8877 9993; fax: 020 8877 9980; website: www.ion.ac.uk.

176. William J. Walsh, Ph.D., "Biochemical Treatment: Medicines for the Next Century," *NOHA (Nutrition for Optimal Health Association) News* 16:3 (Summer 1991), available on the HRI-PTC website (www.hriptc.org/nextcentury.htm). William J. Walsh, Ph.D., "The Critical Role of Nutrients in Severe Mental Symptoms," available on the Internet (www.alternativemental-health.com/articles/article-pffeiffer.htm).

177. Kay Redfield Jamison, *An Unquiet Mind: A Memoir of Moods and Madness* (New York: Knopf, 1995): 6.

6: Amino Acids: Giving the Brain What It Needs

178. Personal communication and Julia Ross, M.A., *The Diet Cure* (New York: Penguin, 1999): 15.

179. *Diet Cure,* 128.

180. Roberto Sanchez, "Actress Urges Better Care for Mentally Ill," *Seattle Times* (April 26, 2000). Available on the Internet at: http://archives.seattletimes.nwsource.com/cgi-bin/texis.cgi/web/vortex/display?slug=kidd26m&date=20000426. *Masks of Madness: Science of Healing,* a film hosted by Margot Kidder; written, produced, and directed by Connie Bortnick; produced in associated with the Canadian Schizophrenia Foundation, 16 Florence Avenue, Toronto, Ontario M2N 1E9 Canada (Sisyphus Communications, Ltd., 1998).

181. From the film *Masks of Madness: Science of Healing,* hosted by Margot Kidder; written, produced, and directed by Connie Bortnick; produced in associated with the Canadian Schizophrenia Foundation, 16 Florence Avenue, Toronto, Ontario M2N 1E9 Canada (Sisyphus Communications, Ltd., 1998).

182. Merrily Manthey, M.S., "Getting Patients Well Is the New Goal of County Treatment Programs," available on the Internet at www.margotkidder.com.

183. From the film *Masks of Madness: Science of Healing,* hosted by Margot Kidder; written, produced, and directed by Connie Bortnick; produced in associated with the Canadian Schizophrenia Foundation, 16 Florence Avenue, Toronto, Ontario M2N 1E9 Canada (Sisyphus Communications, Ltd., 1998).

184. Julia Ross, M.A., *The Diet Cure* (New York: Penguin, 1999): 120.

185. Adapted from: Julia Ross, M.A., *The Diet Cure* (New York: Penguin, 1999): 120–121.

186. From the film *Masks of Madness: Science of Healing,* written, produced, and directed by Connie Bortnick, produced in associated

with the Canadian Schizophrenia Foundation, 16 Florence Avenue, Toronto, Ontario M2N 1E9 Canada (Sisyphus Communications, Ltd., 1998).

187. "New Evidence Points to Opioids," *Autism Research Review International* 5:4 (1991).

188. Paul Shattock, "Urinary Peptides and Associated Metabolites in the Urine of People with Autism Spectrum Disorders," syllabus material for the main DAN! lecture at the DAN! (Defeat Autism Now!) 2000 Conference, in the conference booklet: 79-83; published by the Autism Research Institute in San Diego, Calif. (fax: 619-563-6840 or website: www.autism.com/ari). "New Evidence Points to Opioids," *Autism Research Review International* 5:4 (1991). A. J. Wakefield, et al., "Ileal-Lymphoid-Nodular Hyperplasia, Non-Specific Colitis, and Pervasive Developmental Disorder in Children," *Lancet* 351 (February 28, 1998): 637–41.

189. C. Hallert, et al., "Psychic Disturbances in Adult Coeliac disease III. Reduced Central Monoamine Metabolism and Signs of Depression," *Scand J Gastroenterol* 17 (1982): 25–8.

190. Ron Hoggan, M.A., and James Braly, M.D., "How Modern Eating Habits May Contribute to Depression," available on the Internet at: http://depression.about.com/library/weekly/aa071299.htm.

191. See Depression: Causes (Food Allergies/Intolerances) at http://www.yournutrition.co.uk/specific_health_problems_D.htm.

192. Adapted from: Karyn Seroussi, *Unraveling the Mystery of Autism and Pervasive Developmental Disorder*, New York: Simon & Schuster, 2000: 229–30.

7: Restoring the Tempo of Health: Cranial Osteopathy

193. Stephanie Marohn, *The Natural Medicine Guide to Autism* (Charlottesville, Va.: Hampton Roads, 2002): chapter 8.

194. "What Is Osteopathy?" available at the Cranial Academy website (http://www.cranialacademy.org/whatis.html).

195. H.I. Magoun, D.O., *Osteopathy in the Cranial Field*, 3d Ed., Kirksville, Mo.: Journal Printing Company, 1976: 1.

196. "What Is Osteopathy?" available at the Cranial Academy Website (http://www.cranialacademy.org/whatis.html).

197. "Common Problems," available at the Cranial Academy Website (http://www.cranialacademy.org/cmpr.html).

198. Marohn, *Autism*, chapter 8.

199. Ibid.

200. Lawrence Lavine, "Osteopathic and Alternative Medicine Aspects of Autistic Spectrum Disorders," article on the Internet (available at http://trainland.tripod.com/lawrencelavine.htm).

201. Marohn, *Autism*, chapter 9.

202. Marohn, *Autism,* chapter 8.

8: Bipolar Disorder and Allergies: NAET

203. Devi S. Nambudripad, D.C., L.Ac., R.N., Ph.D., *Say Goodbye to Illness*, New & Revised ed. (Buena Park, Calif.: Delta Publishing, 1999) 35.

204. Devi S. Nambudripad, D.C., L.Ac., R.N., Ph.D., *Say Goodbye to Allergy-Related Autism* (Buena Park, Calif.: Delta Publishing, 1999) 32–47.

205. Nambudripad, *Illness*, 296.

206. Nambudripad, *Illness*, xxii.

207. Personal communication with Dr. Nambudripad, 2001. Richard Leviton, "The Allergy-Free Body," *Alternative Medicine Digest* 6 (April 1995): 13.

208. Nambudripad, *Illness*, xxiii.

209. Reprinted by permission of Devi S. Nambudripad, D.C., L.Ac., R.N., Ph.D., from her book *Say Goodbye to Illness*, New & Revised ed. (Buena Park, Calif.: Delta Publishing, 1999): 366–8.

210. Nambudripad, *Illness*, 147–8.

211. Richard Leviton, "The Allergy-Free Body," *Alternative Medicine Digest* 6 (April 1995): 8.

212. Nambudripad, *Illness*, 33.

9: Rebalancing the Vital Force: Homeopathy

213. Personal communication, 2001. Unless footnoted, quotes throughout this section are from personal communication with Dr. Reichenberg-Ullman.

214. Personal communication, and Judyth Reichenberg-Ullman, N.D., L.C.S.W., and Robert Ullman, N.D., *Prozac Free: Homeopathic Alternatives to Conventional Drug Therapies* (Berkeley, Calif.: North Atlantic Books, 2002): xiv.

215. *Prozac Free,* viii, ix.

216. *Prozac Free,* xiv.

217. Miranda Castro, R. S. Hom., *The Complete Homeopathy Handbook* (New York: St. Martin's Press, 1990): 3–5. Anne Woodham and David Peters, M.D., *Encyclopedia of Healing Therapies* (New York: Dorling Kindersley, 1997): 126.

218. Judyth Reichenberg-Ullman, N.D., M.S.W., and Robert Ullman, N.D., *Ritalin-Free Kids: Safe and Effective Homeopathic Medicine for ADHD, and Other Behavioral and Learning Problems* (Roseville, Calif.: Prima Health, 2000): 83.

219. *Ritalin-Free Kids,* 95.

220. *Ritalin-Free Kids,* 95–6.

221. Personal communication and *Ritalin-Free Kids,* 90.

222. Personal communication and *Prozac Free,* 57.

10: The Shamanic View of Mental Illness

223. John Lash, *The Seeker's Handbook* (New York: Harmony Books, 1990): 371.

224. Holger Kalweit, "When Insanity Is a Blessing," in Stanislav Grof, M.D., and Christina Grof, eds., *Spiritual Emergency* (New York: Jeremy P. Tarcher/Putnam, 1989): 80.

225. Jan Fawcett, M.D., Bernard Golden, Ph.D., and Nancy Rosenfeld, *New Hope for People with Bipolar Disorder* (Roseville, Calif.: Prima, 2000): 296.

226. Richard Leviton, *The Healthy Living Space* (Charlottesville, Va.: Hampton Roads, 2001): 354–8.

227. Ibid, 362–3.

228. Ibid, 364.

229. Malidoma Patrice Somé, *Ritual: Power, Healing, and Community* (New York: Penguin, 1997): 12, 19.

230. Malidoma Patrice Somé, *Of Water and the Spirit: Ritual, Magic, and Initiation in the Life of an African Shaman* (New York: Penguin, 1994): 9, 10.

Conclusion

231. P. Stokes and A. Holtz, "Fluoxetine Tenth Anniversary Update: the Progress Continues," *Clinical Therapeutics* 19:5 (1997): 1135–250.

232. C. Murray and A. Lopez, eds., *The Global Burden of Disease: A Comprehensive Assessment of Mortality and Disability from Diseases, Injuries, and Risk Factors in 1990 and Projected to 2020* (Cambridge: Harvard University Press, 1996).

Index

About the Author

Stephanie Marohn has been writing since she was a child. Her adult writing background is extensive in both journalism and nonfiction trade books. In addition to *Natural Medicine First Aid Remedies* and the six books in the Healthy Mind series (*The Natural Medicine Guide to Autism, The Natural Medicine Guide to Depression, The Natural Medicine Guide to Bipolar Disorder, The Natural Medicine Guide to Addiction, The Natural Medicine Guide to Anxiety,* and *The Natural Medicine Guide to Schizophrenia*), she has published over thirty articles in magazines and newspapers, written two novels and a feature film screenplay, and has had her work included in poetry, prayer, and travel writing anthologies.

Originally from Philadelphia, she has been a resident of the San Francisco Bay Area for over twenty years, and currently lives in Sonoma County, north of the city.

Hampton Roads Publishing Company

: . . for the evolving human spirit

HAMPTON ROADS PUBLISHING COMPANY pub-
lishes books on a variety of subjects, including
spirituality, health, and other related topics.

For a copy of our latest trade catalog, call toll-free,
434-296-2772, or send your name and address to:

HAMPTON ROADS PUBLISHING COMPANY, INC.
PO BOX 8107 • CHARLOTTESVILLE, VA 22906
e-mail: hrpc@hrpub.com • www.hrpub.com